The Health Babes'
GUIDE TO BALANCING HORMONES

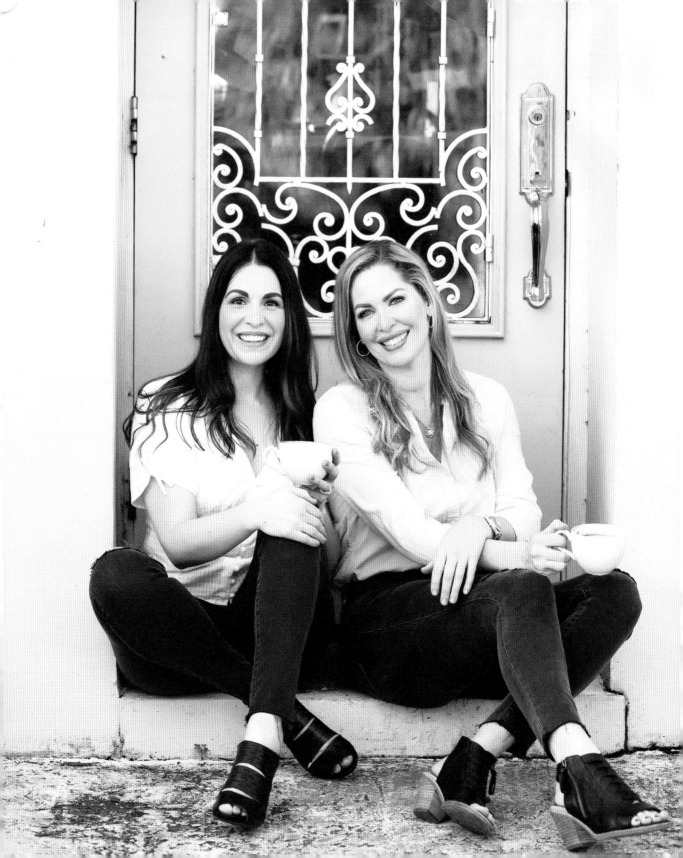

The Health Babes'
GUIDE TO BALANCING HORMONES

A Detailed Plan with Recipes to Support Mood,
Energy Levels, Sleep, Libido and More

DR. KRYSTAL HOHN AND DR. BECKY CAMPBELL

Hosts of The Health Babes podcast

PAGE STREET
PUBLISHING CO.

PAGE STREET
PUBLISHING CO.

First published in 2022 by

Page Street Publishing Co.

27 Congress Street, Suite 1511

Salem, MA 01970

www.pagestreetpublishing.com

Distributed by Macmillan, sales in Canada by The Canadian Manda Group.

26 25   24   23   22   1 2   3 4 5

ISBN-13: 978-1-64567-671-3

ISBN-10: 1-64567-671-4

Library of Congress Control Number: 2022940373

Cover and book design by Meg Baskis for Page Street Publishing Co.

Photography by Becky Campbell

Printed and bound in the United States

Dedication

This book is dedicated to everyone who has decided that they will not accept answers like, "It's just your age," "It's all in your head" or anything along those lines, as an answer to the signals your body is sending you.

Congratulations on deciding to listen to your body and learn about how to best support your health and feel your best. We are honored that you are putting your health in our hands and hope to give you all the answers you need.

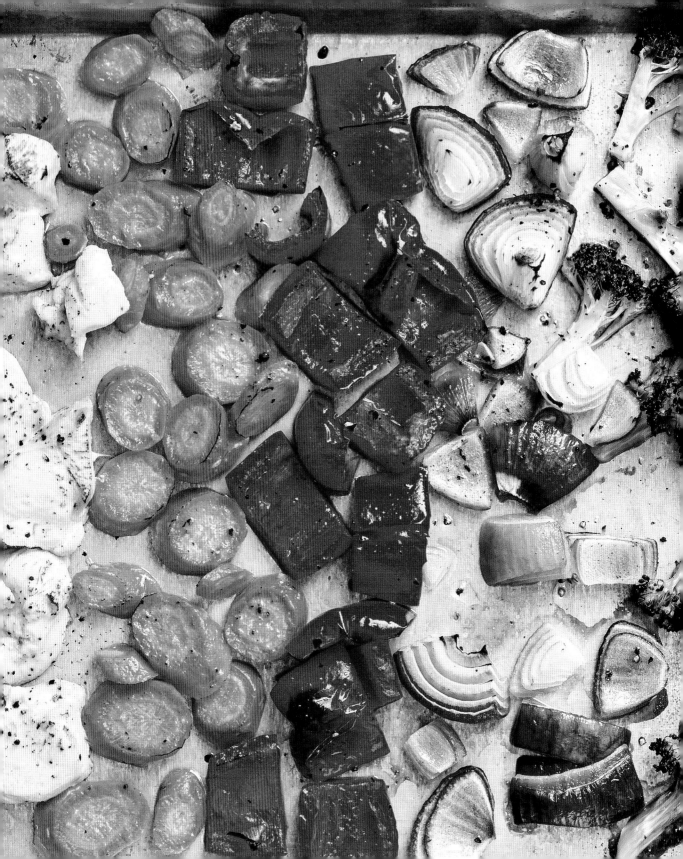

Contents

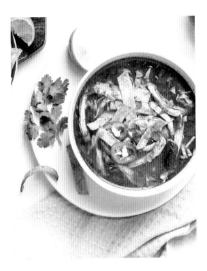

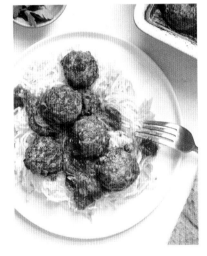
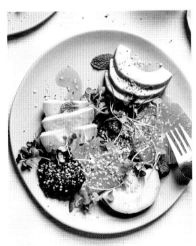

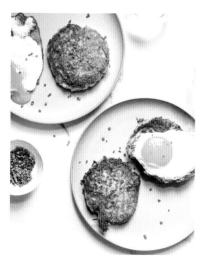

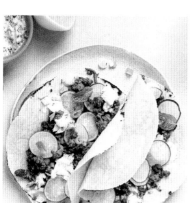

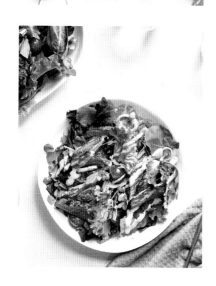

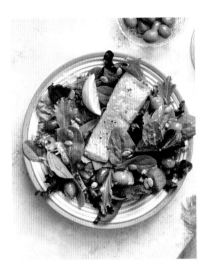

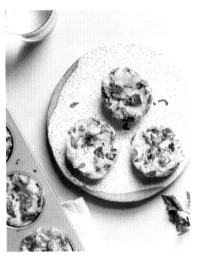

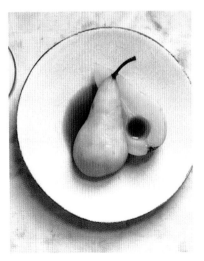

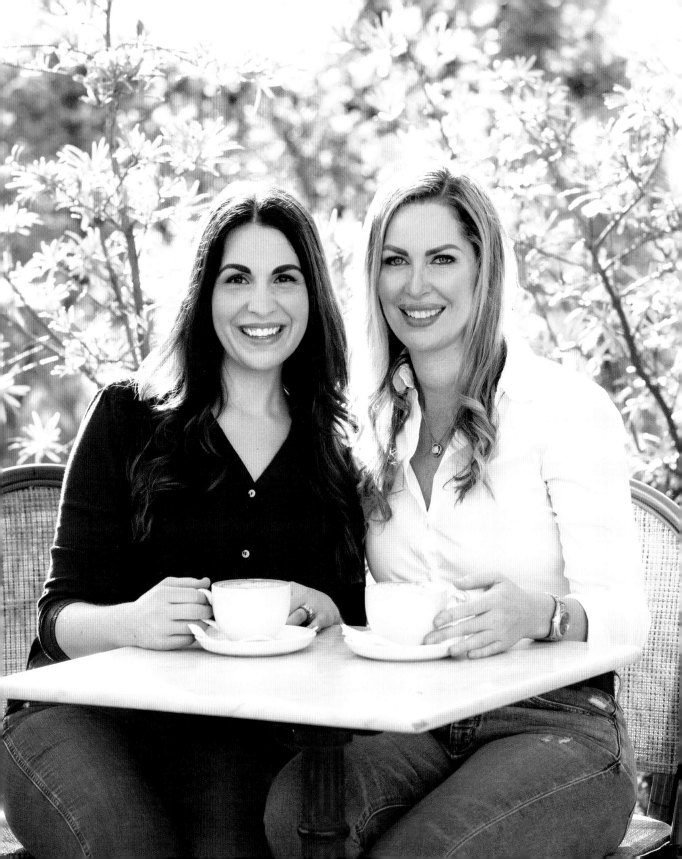

INTRODUCTION: OUR STORY

If you know anything about us, you know that we both struggled with our own health issues for years before figuring out what was causing them. The thing is, all health issues have a root cause. The problem with that is most people don't know where to even begin or who to turn to when figuring this out. Between the two of us, we have had thyroid issues, estrogen dominance, androgen dominance, histamine intolerance, adrenal hormone imbalance—the list goes on.

So, trust us when we tell you . . . we get it. We get how painful this can all be and how frustrating it is when no one understands or takes your health issues seriously. This is the exact reason we do what we do. We want to fill you with as much knowledge as we can on how the body works so that you too can get better, the way that we both have.

Dr. Becky's Story

I want you to know that functional medicine practitioners were usually patients that could not find answers to their health issues before they became a practitioner. I am a practitioner who has been in your shoes and has been down the modern medical route time and time again with disappointment. This is why I am passionate about what I do, because I can relate to almost every one of my patients and readers on a personal level.

I know how hard it is to be sick and tired of feeling sick and tired, and feeling like no doctor can give you an answer. This is why it's my mission to help you uncover your own personal root cause with each book I write.

So here is my story, and how I went from being sick to finding my root cause and eventually putting all of my symptoms into remission. I believe that it sets the tone for the book—that there is hope and feeling better is possible. I offer this inspiration to help you move forward towards uncovering your root causes and encourage you to keep advocating for your health.

For as long as I can remember, I have never felt good. I remember being younger and wanting to go home from school because I was tired or just didn't feel well. In high school, I missed a lot of my early morning classes because I couldn't get out of bed on time. I remember being so fatigued, and it seemed like I was the only one who was dealing with this. No one else around me seemed to have any of the same issues. While I was trying to get through high school, I was also trying to figure out why I felt so exhausted all of the time.

Fast forward to graduate school where I had an enormous amount of stress, barely any time to eat and was working out way too hard for the amount of calories I was taking in. I started getting extreme anxiety, debilitating brain fog, my hair was falling out in clumps and I gained thirty pounds very quickly, despite working out 6 days a week. I also suffered with migraine headaches, strange crawling sensations on my scalp, food sensitivities, abdominal bloating— the list goes on.

It wasn't until I found a holistic health practitioner that I learned why all of this was happening to me. I was finally diagnosed with Hashimoto's thyroiditis, gut infections, high cortisol (stress hormone), estrogen dominance, mercury toxicity, chronic EBV, and about 10 years later, I would diagnose myself with something called Mast Cell Activation Syndrome and Histamine Intolerance.

I want to teach you about root cause(s) because this is how you heal your body.

Dr. Krystal's Story

Most of us start in functional medicine because we know what it's like to feel badly. When I found what worked for me, I wanted to share it with others.

As long as I can remember, I suffered from bloating, IBS and anxiety. As a kid, I would constantly have a stomachache or get ear infections. Fast forward to graduate school when stress was high; my anxiety and gut symptoms were exacerbated. This is when I started diving into nutrition. I was researching inflammatory foods and the impact they had on my gut health. After removing a lot of these foods, I started feeling better.

Later on, after I had my son, I really started to feel off. I could tell my hormones were dysregulated. The lack of sleep, feeling isolated in motherhood and the stress of owning a business was really weighing on me. I was gaining weight, developing cystic acne and felt like I was crawling out of my skin. I can remember canceling events because my skin was so inflamed. Not only did I feel badly on the inside, I was so insecure about how I looked on the outside too. Through functional medicine, I soon found out that I was dealing with estrogen dominance, high testosterone and a candida gut infection that was contributing to a lot of my symptoms.

I worked on my gut, spent time on stress management and eliminated foods that were contributing to my imbalances.

My skin soon cleared, I felt energized, lost weight and my gut symptoms started to melt away.

The experience with my hormones is what led me to my passion for writing this book, working with patients and creating a health brand. It's the reason why I spend most days in the trenches, guiding patients to health. There is so much disconnection in healthcare today. My hope is that this book helps you understand just how important your hormones are. When your body gives you a symptom, there is a reason behind it. You just have to be open and make the changes to better your health.

How We Started The Health Babes

You know when you meet someone and you just totally get each other? Even if others don't get you, you have a secret bond that no one will ever understand. Welp, that is us! We have known each other for years and attended the same graduate school. We joined forces in our virtual practice, working with people all over the world with a multitude of health issues. However, we wanted to be able to reach more people on a broader level, so we locked arms and The Health Babes brand was born.

We want to empower everyone to take better care of themselves by learning what is driving their health issues, instead of landing at a dead end with other practitioners. We want to provide knowledge that is fun and easy to understand. We wrote this book so that we can give you the tools to help the many hormonal imbalances we see today. We all should have an understanding of how our bodies work and function. When we understand this, we make lasting changes. Our goal for you while reading this book would be to implement the tools we provide, understand how your hormones work and to incorporate healthier, hormone-balancing meals. In our experience, if you do all of these things, you will notice an increase in energy, better sleep, increased libido, weight loss, improved skin, better digestion and better mental clarity. Now let's get to work!

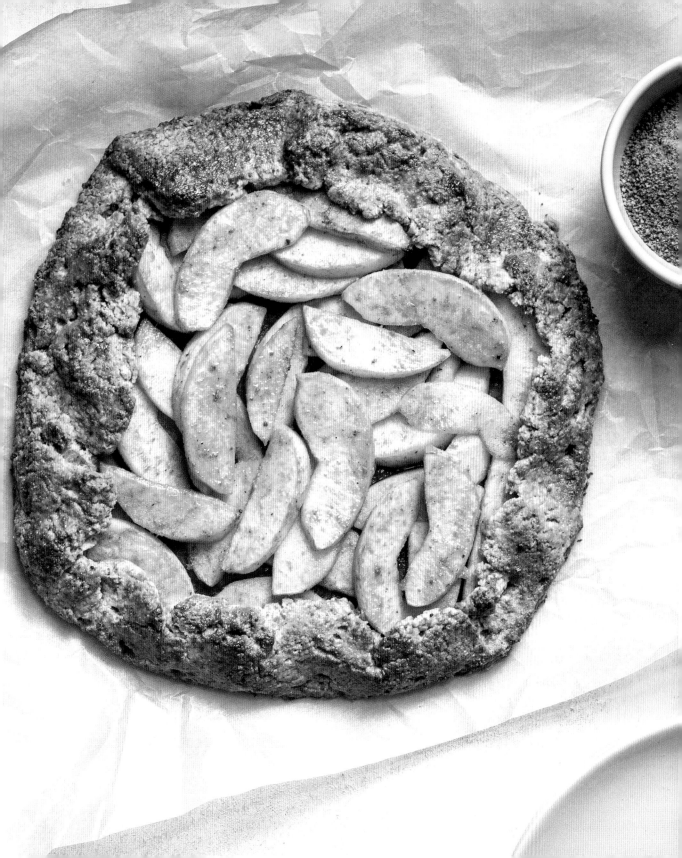

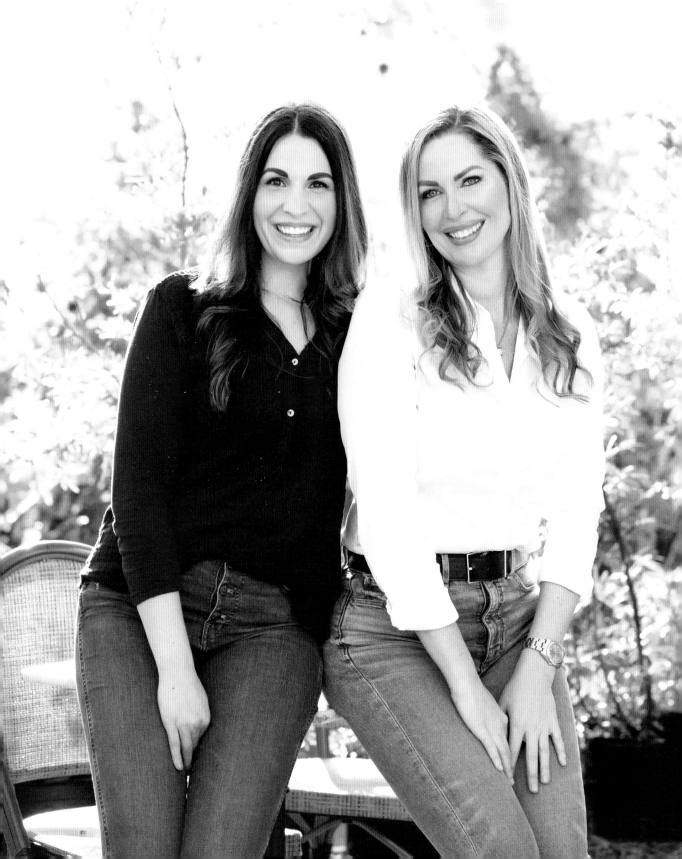

One

AN INTRODUCTION TO HORMONES

What Are Hormones & Why Do They Matter?

When you think of hormones, what comes to mind? Many of you would picture estrogen and testosterone, and some of you might even expand and think about thyroid hormones and cortisol.

You'd be right! Those are all hormones, but there's so much more to discover and explore when it comes to these tiny but powerful chemicals produced by the body—particularly, the multitude of functions they have, over and above just controlling your menstrual cycle (or lack thereof), your weight and your stress levels.

Before we dive into these fascinating intricacies related to hormones, it's important for you to have a little more of an idea of what they really are and why they do what they do. Essentially, what we'd like to achieve is an expansion of what you may already know about hormones and to provide you with a far better understanding of their effects in your own body.

So settle in, grab a hot cuppa tea, and let's begin.

Hormones are chemicals produced by the endocrine glands.

The what glands?

Endocrine simply means that these tissues or glands in the body produce and deliver the chemicals into the bloodstream to be transported via circulation to a site in the body where they will have an impact. This impact is dictated by the type of receptor on the site. Now, a receptor is basically the part of a tissue or cell that is made specifically for the hormone. Essentially, it catches the hormone so that the cell can perform a function.

Picture this: If you wanted to satisfy your thirst, you would pour water into a glass and drink it. If you were to pour water onto the countertop, not only would it go everywhere, but you'd also have a very difficult time trying to satisfy your thirst.

The water in this example is the hormone, the glass the receptor, and when you take a sip, well, that is the action; the water is performing a function, satisfying your thirst.

Don't worry, you're not going to be tested on any of this. Instead, as you read further, this little bit of complex information will allow you to have a better grasp of the good, the bad and the ugly that we're going to talk about, and why the hormone, the receptor and the function are so pertinent to you as an individual and the stage of life you're in.

Now that you know what an endocrine gland is, let's dive in a little deeper. There are nine major endocrine glands, and they are placed strategically throughout the body.

You have the hypothalamus, pituitary gland, pineal gland, thyroid, parathyroids, thymus, pancreas, adrenal glands and ovaries (female) or testes (male).

Even though they are largely separate in where they are, they will all be considered part of the endocrine system (see, another use of the word endocrine— aren't you glad you know what it means?) of course, not only because they all make hormones, but because they have interconnected relationships.

From sleep to temperature control, metabolism, reproduction, stress, infection and more, these hormones and their relationship to one another control almost every cell and organ, telling your body how it is supposed to function.

There are a number of key factors to consider when thinking about the functions that hormones have. It's not just a case of whether the hormone is being produced, but whether it's being produced in the right amount. Upon reading this, many of you may already know that low levels of hormones would cause some serious underperformance issues in your body. But did you know that when hormone levels are too high, it can be just as detrimental? It's true.

Think back to the water in the glass. Not only are you going to stay thirsty if there are just a few drops of water in the glass for you to drink, pouring too much water in the glass is going to leave a big mess for you to clean up before you can even think about having your first sip. Too much of one or more hormones in circulation also causes a mess that your body has to clean up, leaving it less able to concentrate on some other necessary functions.

Worse yet, imagine you didn't have water to fill your glass. Exactly. You'd be thirsty and likely unable to concentrate on much else. The same goes for hormones; a gland that fails to produce a hormone can have serious and negative consequences.

Fortunately, a complete loss of hormone production is not very common. Remember those interconnecting relationships we mentioned earlier? It's the very reason that each gland has a supporting gland to back it up. However, you run the risk of having too little a supply to meet the demand that the body actually needs, as that supporting gland also has its own systems to keep functioning.

Now that you know what hormones are and why they matter, let's talk about the hormones themselves.

The Hormonal Chain of Command

Quiz time!

Without Googling the answer, how many hormones do you think there are in the human body?

Five? Ten? Maybe Twenty?

Many of you will likely be surprised to learn that there are actually fifty, yes, a whopping fifty hormones in humans, all working to keep your body running as it should.

We aren't—some of you may say, fortunately—going to go into each one of these and their functions . . . for that we'd need many more pages. What we are going to do, however, is detail the most important of the fifty, and touch on some of the others that may also be pertinent to their role.

There are seven important hormones we'll get into. These really are part of the nitty gritty, day-to-day hormones that you'll know all about when they're out of whack:

1. ESTROGEN

As your breasts started to develop, you noticed hairs sprouting in places you'd never had them before, and when you had your first menstrual cycle, you were introduced to estrogen.[1] While estrogen is the hormone that gives women their female characteristics, men have a small amount of estrogen, too.

Estrogen, which is mainly made by the ovaries, but supported by the adrenal glands, is actually a blanket name for three different hormones: estradiol, estrone and estriol. Estradiol, also called E^2, is the most potent form of the three, and is prominent in women who are still in their childbearing years. Estrone, on the other hand, or E^1, is the hormone you'll become more familiar with when your menstrual cycle stops and you have gone through menopause. Lastly, estriol or E^3, is mainly produced during pregnancy.

Estrogen levels fluctuate in a cyclical fashion throughout the month. The more dramatic the change in its levels, the more you'll notice. Did anyone say PMS? That's right! Estrogen is responsible for tender breasts, water retention, cravings, heightened emotional responses and those lovely spots that pop up on our skin at certain times of the month.

In the next chapters, we'll be talking a lot more about this hormone, not only when things go wrong, but why. So keep reading!

2. PROGESTERONE

If you talk about estrogen, you simply have to talk about progesterone. While estrogen gets a lot of the credit as it is preparing your body to be able to have a baby, progesterone is the hormone that actually enables you to make a human being.

As you go into your luteal phase of menstruation—essentially the second half of your cycle after ovulation, which we'll discuss more in depth in later chapters—progesterone levels released by the ovaries begin to rise. Should a sperm fertilize an egg, progesterone steals the show, helping that little egg (now called a zygote) embed into now thickened uterine tissue. Progesterone helps to prepare the uterus to continue to nurture a now growing fetus.[2]

If no fertilization or implantation takes place, that thickened lining is useless, so the body gets rid of it. Along with a drop in progesterone, the body sheds the uterine lining, and hello period.

More about this later . . .

3. TESTOSTERONE

Testosterone is the predominant hormone in the male body. It is responsible for a lot of traits such as facial hair, muscle growth, sex drive, temperament, bone mass and production of sperm, to name a few. Too much of a good thing and it can turn ugly, which you'll discover in a bit.[3]

While predominantly a male-pattern hormone, in much smaller amounts, testosterone contributes to women's health too, and you'll come to find out that it can also cause severe problems when it is out of whack.

4. DHEA

We don't hear much about DHEA until there's a reason . . . which is unfortunate, as it's not only a precursor to your sex hormones, but it's also the one that's produced in the largest amounts. Of course, its power is only really known when it becomes one of the other sex hormones, but it's important to mention nonetheless.[4]

When the body needs more estrogen, progesterone or testosterone to be made, signals in the brain tell DHEA, produced by the ovaries or testes, to get to work.

In later chapters you'll discover why problems can arise when DHEA doesn't behave like it should.

5. THYROID HORMONES

How many times have you used the phrase, "Oh, my metabolism is so slow"? While we often link metabolism solely to weight loss and gain in terms of how the body uses food, it's so much more than that. You really can't think about your metabolism without thinking about the thyroid and how the hormones it produces control every energy-using or metabolic cell in your body.[5]

Producer of the four "T" hormones, T3 and T4 being the most important, the thyroid controls everything from your weight to energy levels, how your body manages temperature changes, brain function, bone health, growth and so much more.

6. INSULIN

You probably have a love-hate relationship with insulin and don't even know it. It's essentially the hormone that tells your cells to use up blood sugar or send it for storage.[6] Yup, good old insulin that's produced by the pancreas can dictate whether you're high on energy, using your carbs as fuel or feeling sluggish and not fitting into your favorite pair of jeans.

Insulin is a very interesting hormone that we'll be sure to get more into in a bit!

Cortisol is your main stress hormone. Any stressful event, whether it's physical or psychological, will send signals from the hypothalamus and pituitary glands in your brain to tell your adrenal glands (situated right at the top of each kidney) to release cortisol. It's an important pathway in the stress response known as the HPA axis (hypothalamic-pituitary-adrenal axis).

Cortisol helps to direct the most important resources, namely oxygen-rich blood and blood sugar, to the muscles and tissues that need it most in order to run away from danger or be able to stay and fight. This is known as the fight or flight response.[7] Cortisol further redirects these resources away from the body systems that aren't critical to life. If you have to confront someone in a dark alleyway, the last thing your body needs is to focus on digestive function or reproduction, but you sure do need your eyes to see clearly, your thoughts to be rational and your muscles to be ready for whatever may come your way.

While you may think that you need to stop cortisol from being produced in order to prevent adverse effects associated with high levels, cortisol really offers a protective function to the body when it is produced at the appropriate times and at the appropriate level. This is why cortisol raises your blood sugar, dilates your pupils and slows down digestion when an intense situation arises. After this passes, your body should bring your cortisol back to normal levels and reset blood sugar, digestion and other functions to baseline.

When we are under chronic stress, we do not return back to baseline as we should. This is when you start to see problems arise such as high blood sugar, weight gain, insomnia and a slew of other symptoms.

In later chapters, we'll discuss more about how highs and lows affect other body systems and can leave you feeling anything but well. We'll also touch on the complementary hormone, adrenaline, as it is also involved in the fight or flight response.

The Traveling Trio & the Stages of Your Menstrual Cycle

With a far better understanding of the hormones you have in your body, we can now get into a little more detail about how their levels change depending on the phase of life you are in.

In this section, it's all about *that* time of the month: your period. So, what do we know about menstruation?

Well, for one, some love it and many absolutely hate it, but we all know that it has one important purpose: reproduction. That's right ladies, no period, no babies.

As we dive deeper into the menstrual cycle and all of the intricate processes that take place during the various phases, we're certain you'll come to greatly appreciate your cycle as the fascinating rhythm it is.

Let's get the basics out of the way.

A cycle is basically a sequence of events that take place in a given period of time, and then starts all over again. The menstrual cycle is typically around 28 days for many women, but anything from 21 to 35 days can be considered normal.[8] For the purpose of explaining the menstrual cycle and what happens during each phase, we'll be referring to a 28-day cycle.

Now comes the fun part: the phases.

There are two phases in the menstrual cycle:[9] the follicular phase and the luteal phase. The follicular phase kicks off right after menstruation and the two phases are then neatly divided by ovulation around the middle of the cycle. In a 28-day cycle,[10] the follicular phase lasts around 10 to 16 days, ovulation around 1 day, the luteal phase around 14 days and your period or bleeding time around 4–7 days. These phases are really controlled by changes in hormone levels that dictate what happens during your period.

What we're going to get into now are the hormones, and keep in mind that this is going to be largely dictated by a regular 28-day cycle. We promise that the trouble you typically face as a result of hormone fluctuations throughout the menstrual cycle will come later, but for now, we stick to learning the basics.

There are three main hormone role players in the menstrual cycle: the trio, if you will. They are estrogen, progesterone and testosterone. Testosterone? A male hormone? Regulating the menstrual cycle? It's true! Remember back to the beginning of this book where you learned that testosterone was also produced in smaller amounts in women? Well, this hormone has a bigger role than you thought, and you'll discover why in just a bit.

First up, however, is the role of estrogen and progesterone.

During the follicular phase,[11] the ovaries start to make between five and twenty follicles, each of which will carry an egg. This process is largely guided by another hormone, called the follicle stimulating hormone (FSH). Initially, estrogen and progesterone remain relatively low during this stage, but as the follicles develop and mature as the days go by, estrogen levels start to rise while progesterone remains at a trickle. Estrogen helps to thicken and prepare the lining of the uterus to become a cozy and nourishing bed for a fertilized egg to embed into.

Estrogen then continues to rise, which signals the major endocrine gland in the brain called the pituitary gland. It releases a hormone called the luteinizing hormone (LH), and it's a huge spike of available LH that triggers ovulation, which is the release of the dominant egg from one of the matured follicles.

Let's get back to testosterone for a minute. You'll likely find it interesting that this hormone may, along with estrogen, prepare the uterus for implantation and help prepare it to support pregnancy. It too has a little spike, along with estrogen production, at the time of ovulation. It's this brief surge in testosterone around ovulation that increases libido.[12] Hey, what's better for the chances of implantation of that ready-than-ever-egg than a naturally heightened sex drive? Nature is incredible, isn't it?

Back to the phases of the cycle!

Following the 24-hour ovulation period is the start of the luteal phase. It's during this stage that the body has to make some important decisions. Does it continue to support the growth of the endometrial lining or does it allow it to shed, ready for the next cycle to start? This all hangs on one thing: was the egg fertilized or not?

There's a critical and narrow window in which implantation can take place. That little mature egg only has 24 hours to survive traveling down the fallopian tubes, looking for an easy-to-please sperm. Fortunately, sperm *can* stay active for up to 5 days after unprotected sex, which leaves the chances of fertilization far more probable than relying on a single 24-hour window in which the egg is viable.

Now, during this time following ovulation, progesterone starts to go from a trickle to a full-blown waterfall[13]—all in an effort to ensure things are well and ready for implantation and to be prepared to support the vulnerable egg should it be fertilized. Estrogen also continues to climb, as does the growth of the uterine lining.

Without fertilization, however, there is no need to support the cozy environment where a fetus may begin to grow. Instead, progesterone and estrogen begin to decline, and when they reach their lowest levels, that's when menses takes place. It's the decline in estrogen and progesterone without implantation that triggers the body to get rid of what is not needed, and so the thickened uterine lining starts to shed. Days later, it all starts again.

That's really the most important part of the menstrual cycle. Fascinating.

Bringing Sexy Back . . . Wait, I Think I Lost It: Welcome to Perimenopause

When you're in the prime time of your reproductive years, the regularity of your cycles and estrogen levels are largely under the control of the two hormones that are released during the follicular and luteal phases of your cycle, namely FSH and LH. As your reproductive window begins to close, there's little need to continue the hard work involved in preparing the body for implantation of a fertilized egg and you begin to transition into perimenopause.

The most common signs that one is in perimenopause are associated with changes in body temperature that may cause you to wake up in the middle of the night with sweats or experience those hot rushes that seem to last for hours and come on in the most inappropriate of times, along with low libido and periods that go all out of whack.

Good question, and to tell you the truth, perimenopause, what it is and what actually takes place in the body seems to be a cause of much confusion, even in the highly specialized world of medicine. For centuries, the main concern was menopause itself, and poor old perimenopause was the girl left in the corner at the dance, being paid little attention.

You see, with menopause, we would look at a *drop* in the levels of hormones as an indication of the transition, and along with it all of the corresponding symptoms associated with lower hormone levels, which you're absolutely right about, are hot flashes, night sweats and low libido.

After a little more research, and to be honest, giving perimenopause a little more well-deserved attention, we're now much smarter and far wiser, and we know that one of the earliest features of perimenopause is a *spike* in estrogen production. And even a *rise* in estrogen, not only a drop, can cause these symptoms.[14]

Interestingly, research shows that levels can climb as much as 30 percent as you go through perimenopause. Along with the surge comes a few unwanted side effects, which you may be all too familiar with, as you likely also experienced them as you were going through your regular menstrual cycle when you were younger and you had estrogen spikes around ovulation and the start of your cycle. Some of the awful symptoms you may experience include breast tenderness, bloating, irregular cycles that can flood when they do come, irritability, mood swings, headaches, weight gain, hair loss, sleeping issues, brain fog, anxiety . . . oh boy!

And don't forget—now we know that sweats and hot flashes, as well as little interest in sex, can be added to the list.

Do you want to know why this rollercoaster ride of estrogen takes place? It's literally the body's last-ditch effort to procreate. We kid you not. With the number of follicles that your ovaries are able to produce on the steep decline, more FSH is needed to get those follicles ready for potential implantation.[15] With a surge in FSH, there's a corresponding surge in stimulation of the ovary. Irritable ovaries are never a good thing, and in this case, they begin to release more estrogen.[16]

If it wasn't bad enough already, there's usually a corresponding decline in the ability to produce enough progesterone, which places additional stress on your body's ability to maintain a sense of hormonal balance. Lowered progesterone levels are associated with shortened luteal phase lengths, which causes ovulation to be skipped.

This growing ratio that separates estrogen and progesterone production makes those high estrogen symptoms even more pronounced. Additionally, higher estrogen sends out stress signals to the brain, which are another reason mood swings and nervous system symptoms such as irritability and anxiety may be far more likely during perimenopause.[17]

Of course, there are many cases where women don't see a significant change in their progesterone levels early on in perimenopause. These are often women who wouldn't have as many dramatic symptoms during this time, but may only start to experience them during menopause as their progesterone levels tend to drop off at that time.

It's for this very reason that each of you reading this book will have a slightly different story to tell once you've gone through perimenopause. Some may experience hot flashes and nighttime sweats, others may not. You may be someone who doesn't have one bothersome symptom, while your bestie is plagued by everyday troubles. Periods may be heavy or light, continue for 3 to 4 years, end in a short few months or even last up to a decade. It really is such an individualized experience based on what your cycles and hormone levels were like before, and your genetics may even play a role.

These reasons are also why it is extremely difficult to tell when exactly you're going to go through perimenopause. Some evidence suggests it's around forty. Other bodies of research suggest it can be as early as in your late thirties. Others still suggest the range is far greater, with perimenopause being able to start taking place in anyone between the ages of thirty-five and sixty.[18]

So, if you don't know when you're going to go through perimenopause, or whether you're in it already, here are some of the defined characteristics; being positive for any three of these may mean you're in perimenopause.

1. Your menstruation has become heavier and/or longer than it usually was.

2. Your cycle length has become shorter than 25 days.

3. Your breasts have recently become more sore, swollen and/or feel lumpy.

4. Menstrual cramps are a new symptom, or they have become more intensified.

5. A new symptom of mid-sleep waking has emerged.

6. You're waking up with night sweats, especially around the time of menses.

7. A new symptom is migraine headaches, or your current headaches have intensified.

8. You are experiencing a new onset of premenstrual mood swings, or your mood swings have become intensified.

9. You're noticing weight gain without having changed anything in your food intake or exercise routine.

Perimenopause Signs & Symptoms You May Experience

Longer or heavier menstrual cycle

Menstrual cycle length shorter than 25 days

Sore or tender breasts

Menstrual cramps are a new symptom, or they have become more intensified

Waking in the middle of the night

Night sweats

Migraines or intensified headaches

New onset of mood swings, or current mood swings are more intense

Weight gain without having changed anything in your food intake or exercise routine

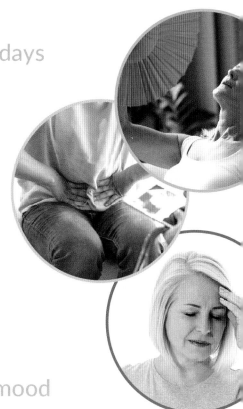

Sexy, Please Don't Leave the Building: Menopause

Let me guess . . . you're around the age of fifty-two, you've been having whirlwind ups and downs with your cycles over the last few years, and now you've been without any inkling of a cycle for at least 12 months?

Yup, it's safe to say, you're in menopause.

While some of you may be celebrating, having finally stopped the rollercoaster ride you've been on with PMS, mood swings and cramps, the thought of menopause may send shivers up your spine. Whichever side of the fence you're sitting on, it's important to address. More important, however, is to educate you about what is considered normal and what is not.

In this section we're looking at you, menopause. And while it doesn't paint a pretty picture right up front, bear with us; this is just the darker side, and we will eventually get into the light when we start looking at the wonderful ways we can support these hormonal changes.

Get cozy, and let's begin.

As you've come to understand, your hormones and ovarian functions control your menstrual cycle, supporting the development of those little egg-containing follicles, allowing the egg to be released during ovulation, and then shedding that prepared uterine lining should the egg not be implanted or fertilized.

Once the ovaries have taken it upon themselves to decide that you're no longer in a state to reproduce, they begin to stop making an effort. In most cases, this happens around the age of fifty-two,[19] but the age of menopause can vary greatly depending on many factors, including sociodemographic, lifestyle choices and genetics factors,[20] which is why the age that your mother went through menopause can give you a rough idea of when you should expect to go through it.

It's at this time that the ovaries no longer build the follicles, no longer release an egg and no longer change the thickness of the lining of the uterus. There's also a decline in the production of estrogen and progesterone that you have to deal with.

Estrogen may be one of the most influential hormones during menopause, as its decline is largely responsible for the symptoms you may experience during this time of your life.[21] Because estrogen is largely a signaling molecule, one that tells various parts of your body what to do, you guessed it, lower estrogen levels can have profound effects on the function of various other body systems.

For example, lower estrogen availability for your brain and nervous system means you may become more emotional, experience more blips in your memory, continue having hot flashes and night sweats, and even develop anxiety and/or depression.[22]

Sad Vagina

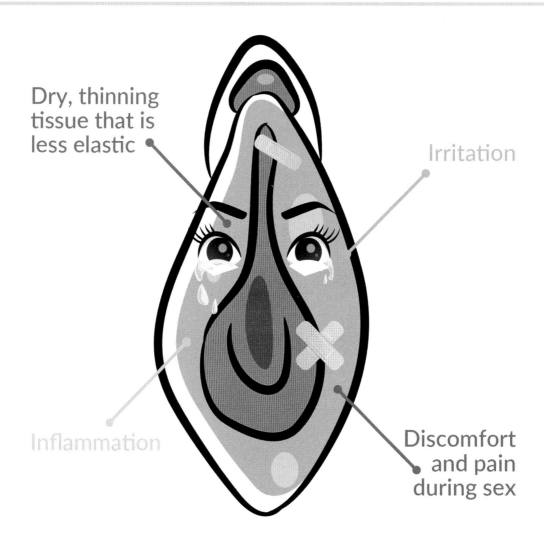

Dry, thinning tissue that is less elastic

Irritation

Inflammation

Discomfort and pain during sex

Low Progesterone Signs & Symptoms

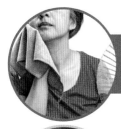 Hot flashes

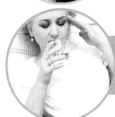 Sleep disturbances

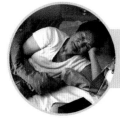 Headaches

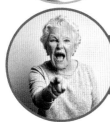 Mood changes

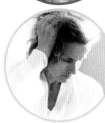 Memory blips

Your urinary tract is also in the line of fire.[25] The tube that transports your urine from your bladder to the toilet becomes thinner and drier. It's less elastic, which means even a little urine in your bladder may escape without you having much control of it doing so. It's also a reason many menopausal women have a higher risk of UTIs because bacteria just love to thrive 'down there,' and these changes give them a far better opportunity to do so.

. . . And your vagina. Your poor vagina. It's subjected to the same fate—dry, thinning tissue that is less elastic. And did we mention dry? Goodbye lubrication and hello irritation, inflammation, discomfort and more pain during sex.[24]

Lower estrogen levels also affect the skin. It's why you feel that your skin is drier, more wrinkles have seemingly sprung up overnight and the crevices are deepening. Your skin feels far thinner, you scratch yourself and it takes absolutely ages to heal, and you start *looking* like you're aging.[25]

Lower levels of progesterone have been implicated in the severity of hot flashes, sleep disturbances, headaches, mood changes and memory blips.[26]

You've also read in the previous chapters that testosterone is the typical hormone that gives you your sex drive. As you get older, it's not just estrogen and progesterone levels that start to dwindle . . . I know what you're thinking . . . OMG, testosterone does too! No wonder the fire you felt for sex is no longer there.[27]

Testosterone is also essential for maintaining muscle and bone mass. That's right! If you're not maintaining testosterone levels, there's little wonder why your bones become frailer (hello, osteoporosis[28]) and you're not as strong as you used to be (struggling to open the jar of pickles all of a sudden?).

It's a sad truth, but testosterone that peaked in your 20s dips to around half of what it was now that you're in menopause. While those little ovaries try to churn out every ounce of testosterone they can despite not producing any estrogen, and the adrenal glands also come to the party with the little they can contribute, it's just not enough.

As you can see, there's a lot the body goes through during this time. It's not all doom and gloom, and many women sail through menopause without so much as a sweat. Keep reading and we'll give you all of the tips and tricks you need to be able to do the same.

Two

THE GOOD, THE BAD, THE UGLY

Hormones need to be made in the right amounts for you to reap their full benefits. High or low simply doesn't cut it and can cause you to experience some awful symptoms as a result.

1) ESTROGEN DOMINANCE: WHEN ESTROGEN LEVELS ARE TOO HIGH

Estrogen keeps us looking and feeling our best. So surely, having more of it would make us feel like we're gorgeous and invincible? We wish! Well, it's not the case, unfortunately. In fact, it's quite the opposite. High estrogen activity due to higher than typical levels flowing through your system spells a range of different health issues.[29]

Research shows that the most common effects resulting from estrogen dominance are diseases such as polycystic ovary syndrome (PCOS) (more on this in the section below) and endometriosis (a condition where the endometrial tissue grows outside of the uterus), as well as breast and ovarian cancer.

Lesser-known effects of estrogen dominance are those on your thyroid and immune system.

High estrogen levels cause the liver to produce a compound called thyroid-binding globulin (TBG). It's a compound that binds to the T3 and T4 hormones, rendering them unavailable to bind to the cells,[30] so you're left feeling less than amazing and fatigued, and you're gaining weight even though you have made no changes to your diet or exercise routine. The thyroid, in response, starts to crank up its production of T3 and T4—after all, these hormones are critical for all metabolic processes in the body. The overtime and hard work is no good for the thyroid and it starts to tire. Hypothyroidism results, and your symptoms worsen over time.

Estrogen can have a serious impact on your immune system, too. We've not only seen estrogen overactivity be associated with autoimmune conditions such as lupus[31] and multiple sclerosis,[32] high levels of estrogen may make a particular type of immune cell, called mast cells, become irritable.[33] Mast cells carry a lot of different compounds around the body. Many of these compounds are responsible for inflammatory conditions; one of these compounds that you may have heard of, is histamine.

High Estrogen Signs & Symptoms

 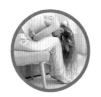

PREMENSTRUAL SYMPTOMS　　**ENDOMETRIOSIS**　　**MENSTRUAL CRAMPS**　　**INFERTILITY**　　**FATIGUE**

    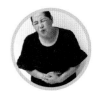

HOT FLASHES　　**DECREASED LIBIDO**　　**HEADACHES**　　**DEPRESSION**　　**EXCESSIVE MENSTRUATION**

 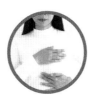

UTERINE FIBROIDS　　**FIBROCYSTIC BREASTS**　　**THYROID ISSUES**　　**BREAST, UTERINE, OVARIAN, PROSTATE, OR COLON CANCER**

Estrogen can bind to the same receptor sites as histamine does (H1 receptors). When this happens, our mast cells release extra histamine, especially in the reproductive organs. Histamine also makes us release more estrogen. So these two work hand in hand to cause the perfect storm.

Why does estrogen go on to dominate? Often, it has to do with lifestyle factors and the inflammation they may cause. Chronic stress, poor gut or liver health, exposure to toxins and poor regulation from the ovaries all play a part. These factors all cause high levels of conversion from androgens, and it floods the body with estrogens. Taking certain medications can also be a problem. Some women develop estrogen dominance from taking the birth control pill or from Metformin (a diabetes drug).

2) ANDROGEN DOMINANCE: WHEN ANDROGEN LEVELS ARE TOO HIGH

The term androgen refers to hormones such as testosterone and DHEA as well as the metabolites that they are broken down into.

While we all need androgens, if they are too high, they can cause a lot of trouble. If you or anyone you know is dealing with chronic acne, dark hair that grows in inappropriate places, weight gain, thinning hair and intolerance to carbohydrates, it's likely that there is an androgen excess.

What causes androgen levels to increase? Typically, it's a problem with either an overproduction by the ovaries, which can happen in PCOS, or more rarely, a problem with the master endocrine gland—the pituitary gland—which leads to an increase in signaling from the brain that increases androgen production. Because androgens are also produced by the adrenal glands, anything that stimulates higher adrenal output potentially increases androgen production with it.

Lifestyle factors also play a role. If you're having trouble managing your insulin levels, or you're insulin resistant, the body makes less of the compound SHBG (sex hormone binding globulin), which is supposed to mop up any excess hormones. Less SHBG means there are more active forms of androgens flowing about and all too eager to bind to the tissues, causing them to perform unfavorable functions.

Hyperandrogenic PCOS is one of the most common endocrine conditions in women of reproductive age.[34] 60% of individuals with PCOS have higher levels of androgens, and this presents health challenges such as obesity, insulin resistance, high cholesterol and liver problems.[35] Additionally, higher testosterone, DHEA and androstenedione, a metabolite of the breakdown of androgens, affect the ovaries. It's for this reason that many people with PCOS have difficulties maintaining regular cycles and ovulation, often making it very difficult for them to get pregnant or maintain a healthy pregnancy.[36]

There are two other organs besides the ovaries and adrenal glands that we need to address in our androgen excess conundrum. Can you guess what they are?

Fat and the skin.

Ok, you might be thinking, "What in the world are we talking about now? How can the fat and skin *produce hormones?*"

Well, you'd be right to question that . . . they don't actually produce the hormones. Instead, they have a more backstage role, which in fact, is just as concerning. They take weaker androgens that may not be quite so bothersome, and they go and turn them into full-blown dominant ones. So you can see why, when you have more fat and more skin to cover it, there may be a compounding of the androgen problem.

3) CORTISOL IMBALANCE: STRESS ADAPTATION IS MORE IMPORTANT THAN HIGHS AND LOWS!

Oh cortisol, cortisol, cortisol. How misunderstood you are . . .

We want to get rid of cortisol, right? *Wrong!* We want to *balance* cortisol and make sure that we have enough when we do need it and we don't have too much when we don't need it. Essentially, cortisol offers a protective element to your everyday function. When you're in danger, cortisol spikes really quickly, allowing you to make a quick decision to either stay and fight off the danger or run away as quickly as your legs will carry you.

When that danger is no longer present, we want the body to quickly turn that cortisol into inactive cortisol, ready in a storage form, cortisone, to be back to the usable form, cortisol, when we need it most.

Looking at cortisol as a measure of chronic stress, we never want to look at it in isolation. It's not a good enough marker on its own to tell us exactly what is going on. We want to see it in relation to another important hormone to see what stress is doing to the body. That other hormone is DHEA.

Now, we mentioned DHEA in the section on androgens above. DHEA is a major hormone, and like cortisol, is made by the adrenal glands. Importantly, DHEA and cortisol have opposing actions, and research shows that DHEA, especially the sulfated form of DHEA, called DHEAs, is associated with stress adaptation.[37] When DHEAs is in higher amounts than cortisol, it shows that the negative effects on the body may be reduced. The normal DHEAs to cortisol ratio we want to see in this case is around 5:1 or 6:1.

Unfortunately, we often see numbers closer to the 1:1 ratio.

What does this mean? Well, it means that stress is likely having a significant effect on the body, that stress adaptation is poor and that trouble is on the horizon.

When cortisol levels creep up enough to match those of DHEAs, and they stay that way, like what happens with chronic stress, we lose out on the protective function of DHEAs, and this can have widespread implications on health. It is associated with decreased central nervous system function, leading to brain inflammation; it can affect mood and lead to depression; it can cause problems with how your muscles function and maintain their shape and mass; it can cause immune dysfunction, insulin resistance and a whole whack of other nasty conditions.[38]

That's why stress is so detrimental to health. Not simply because it forces the body to produce cortisol, but when it forces the body to produce cortisol for too long, it messes with the protective mechanisms that the body has in place.

4) INSULIN & LEPTIN RESISTANCE: TROUBLE ADJUSTING TO THE FOODS YOU'RE EATING

You've all heard about insulin, but do you know what it does further than helping to push the sugar you obtain from the breakdown of ingested carbohydrates into your cells? Firstly, it also helps to send "leftovers" to the liver for additional storage.

When you're sensitive to insulin, your cells use up what blood sugar availability they can. The rest, like we said, goes to the liver.

When you're insulin resistant, your cells no longer listen to what insulin has to say. They essentially go without fuel and starve. Your liver, on the other hand, is all too eager to help out. The liver cells continue to speak insulin's language and take up all of the available blood sugar that you have.

The trouble is, the liver is only so big. When its capacity is full, it doesn't quit taking sugar in, it simply converts it to a different form: fat or, more precisely, triglycerides. This is the major storage form of fat that accumulates around the liver, the organs, your booty, your belly and bingo wings. Not only are your blood sugar levels sky-high, you feel starving because all of your other cells are low in fuel, but you continue to gain weight when you eat because of the liver's role in this process.[39]

Leptin on the other hand is known as one of the major satiety hormones. Leptin tells your brain that it's time to stop eating.[40] What happens with leptin resistance, when the brain becomes resistant to leptin's messages? Of course, there's no off switch to interrupt the pathway of food from the fork to the mouth.

Leptin resistance is more common than you think, and it could be the reason you're doing everything in your power to maintain a healthy body weight, but not seeing any progress from your efforts.

If any of you have a pet kitty, you're going to understand the concept of leptin resistance very well. Call your cat to come over and they continue what they're doing, completely ignoring you or, more likely, they take a stroll in the opposite direction! It's the same with leptin resistance. You're calling for leptin, but your brain is not getting the message, and is doing something else entirely: telling you that you're starving. So, what happens? You continue to feel hungry, even though you have a sufficient supply of energy both in available blood sugar and the storage form, fat.[40]

You see, it's your fat cells that produce leptin. If your brain doesn't get the message that your fat stores are sufficient, then your brain takes on the role to ensure that you're not starving, and in doing so, "forces" you to keep adding to the fat supplies. You eat and eat and never feel satisfied.

As your fuel stores grow, leptin continues to be produced, but the brain is simply unresponsive to its messages and the cycle continues. In addition, because the brain doesn't recognize the surplus energy in storage, it will also reduce your calorie expenditure at rest. Don't go burning extra fuel, says the brain, not realizing that there is more than enough to go around.

Some of the biggest causes of leptin resistance include inflammatory conditions that interfere with the signals the brain is able to recognize and eating too many foods high in fat. That means, what we're doing here, reducing inflammation and improving the diversity and nutritious array of foods you're taking in, is all in an effort to reverse this dramatic effect that leptin resistance has had on your body.

5) THYROID HORMONE IMBALANCE: THE THYROID BEHAVING BADLY

Every metabolic process that takes place in your body is under the control of the hormones your thyroid produces. We often hear of the troubles that occur when there is too little output, i.e., hypothyroidism, and how that causes fatigue, dry skin, constipation, muscle weakness and weight gain as the most common symptoms. Just like too little, too much output by the thyroid gland can be an issue.

While it may sound inviting to have too much of the hormones that keep you energetic and slim, it's not all rainbows and roses. Hyperthyroidism can be costly to your system. While it does mean burning extra calories, most people with hyperthyroidism will suffer from heart palpitations, feelings of anxiety and restlessness, mood swings, sensitivity to heat, sleep issues, thinning hair and digestive upsets that lead to diarrhea.

Again, it's the *optimal* output by the thyroid gland that keeps the body running like a well-oiled machine.

The most common reason for primary hypothyroidism is iodine deficiency,[41] but there is another way the thyroid can be affected. When the disorders of the thyroid are caused by the body's immune system interfering with the production of hormones, it leads to an autoimmune form of thyroiditis. With an underactive thyroid, the condition is called Hashimoto's thyroiditis and Grave's disease when it causes overactive thyroid function.

Women, or as We Like to Say, the Lucky Ones

Women, with all of your power and beauty, there are some challenges you have to face simply because you are . . . a woman.

From starting puberty and having your first period to going through perimenopause and then menopause, there are severe fluctuations in hormone levels across your lifetime that can leave you feeling like a completely different person.

Hormonal fluctuations can be associated with some really nasty side effects and symptoms:

- Heavy periods or periods that happen too frequently
- Cramping and severe pain during ovulation and/or the first days of your cycle
- Headaches or migraines
- Mood swings
- Brain fog
- Fatigue
- Missed periods
- Acne
- Irregular hair growth
- Brittle bones
- Muscle weakness
- Weight gain
- Digestive disorders
- Sleep disturbances
- Low sex drive
- Infertility
- Blood sugar imbalances

If you're plagued by any of these symptoms on a regular basis, it's time to get those hormones checked. Many of these symptoms are associated with treatable conditions such as:

- High or low estrogen production
- High or low progesterone production
- High or low testosterone production
- PCOS
- Endometriosis
- Fibroids
- Perimenopause
- Menopause
- Chronic stress
- Thyroid disorders
- Prediabetes or diabetes

Men, the Actual Lucky Ones

It might surprise you, but men are not immune to hormonal imbalances. With the changing of our environments and contributing lifestyle factors, many people may face the consequences of changing hormone levels; and it's no longer a case of, "Oh, I only have to worry about that when I'm older . . ."– these hormonal imbalances are now affecting far more men in their younger years.

Exposure to higher than typical estrogen levels can cause changes in your body that resemble more female-typical characteristics. You'll experience mood swings, difficulties maintaining a healthy weight, brain fog, fatigue, anxiety and low libido.

Where is all of this estrogen coming from? Some of the main culprits are found[42]:

- In our food and the hormones pumped into animal produce

- In our water and the endocrine-disrupting chemicals and hormones that flow into ground-water[43]

- From exposure to toxins, called xenoestrogens, that mimic estrogen's effect in the body

As estrogen levels dial up, it causes an imbalance in the testosterone ratio. But it's testosterone that gives typical male characteristics, and so it's a no-brainer that when estrogen takes over, these characteristics also begin to fade.

Of course, it is important to mention the changes that take place during the process of aging. After the age of forty, you'll typically start making less progesterone and with it, testosterone levels start to fall. This process may also lead to a form of estrogen dominance, where in addition to the higher exposure of estrogens across your lifetime, it can cause a range of unpleasant symptoms, as noted above. When the estrogens cannot be naturally balanced with testosterone as you age, there's a risk of a whole whack of other symptoms or conditions.[44] Prostate enlargement, osteoporosis, high cholesterol and urinary tract disease may all develop.

Stress can also have a serious impact on men: not just raising the risk of issues such as high blood pressure and cardiovascular disease, but high levels of cortisol can impair progesterone activity, and as a precursor to testosterone, may disrupt your hormonal balance. Again, it's estrogen that usually comes out on top and those nasty symptoms along with it.

Body weight also plays a role in managing the balance of hormones. Fat cells are not only able to store higher amounts of estrogens[45] but they carry more of a specific type of enzyme the body can use to convert testosterone into estrogen. More aromatase means less testosterone and more estrogen availability, leaving you with the same problems.[46]

Clearly, men are not immune to hormonal issues, they're just not as obvious. Think about those hormonal issues we see in women and how it affects them; hot flashes, weight gain, irritability, night sweats . . . they're all obvious and quite unpleasant. When women are on a hormonal roller coaster, they tend to *look* like they are—sorry, ladies! But what can you expect when stress affects estrogen, which affects thyroid hormones, which affects testosterone, which affects blood sugar levels, which affects stress? And the cycle continues over and over and over . . .

. . . And that's why us women like to call men, the "actual lucky ones."

Leptin & Insulin Resistance

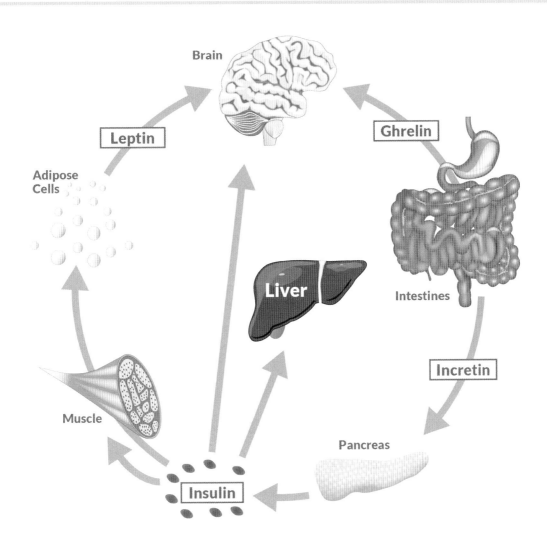

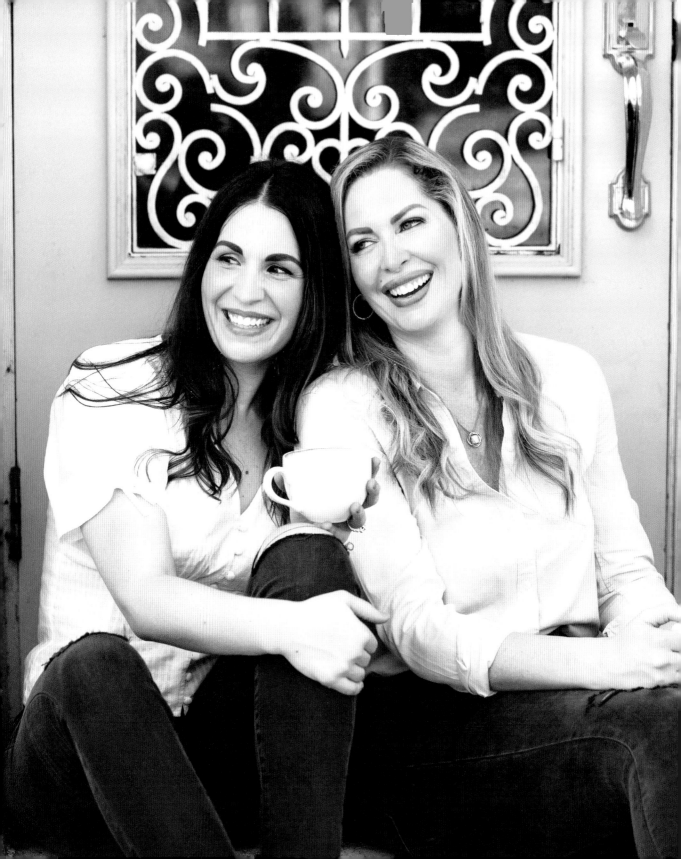

Three

THE TOP FOUR REASONS YOUR HORMONES ARE MISBEHAVING

You've digested no shortage of information pertaining to the hormones and their role in your body. Now we get into the real crux of the matter: why are your hormones not behaving as they should?

If You Didn't Know, Now You Know: The Gut

The gastrointestinal system, a complex system of tissues and organs which is collectively known as the gut, starts in the mouth and ends in the anus. While we know of it fondly as the system that digests foods, absorbs nutrients and eliminates waste, there is so much more to this system that takes up a large portion of the real estate in your body. The gut has input from and influences many other organs and tissues, making it one of *the* top systems to investigate when it comes to hormones and their tendency to misbehave.

More recently, the gut has become a critical area of interest in hormonal balance.[47] Why? Because every system in the body is connected to it in some way or another. For this reason, instead of trying to manage hormones from a single perspective of the production and usage of hormones, we often need to look to the gut for answers, and in particular, what is going on deep within your intestines as the biggest clue.

There are trillions of little critters made up of bacteria, fungi, viruses and other microorganisms known as the microbiota that live in and along your entire digestive tract. Each has their role, but the biggest and most influential colonies live in your large intestine or colon.

A well-functioning gut and microbiota system means that the estrogen balance is well controlled. Some of the species living in the colon produce an enzyme called beta glucuronidase,[48] which breaks estrogens down in the gut after they have been processed by the liver. Dr. Carrie Jones does an amazing job of explaining the three phases of estrogen metabolism (see graph on page 41). This breakdown of estrogens helps with the elimination of estrogens, as the process prevents them from simply being reabsorbed along with other nutrients and reused. But that's the key, isn't it?

If there are not enough of these beta glucuronidase species, or too much estrogen is passing from the liver, estrogens are not being broken down in the gut effectively, and there's a higher risk of them being snapped right back up into the blood and circulation.

Another problem is gut inflammation. When the gut is inflamed, it requires a huge amount of resources to keep functioning as it should. Out of interest, the usual turnaround of cells in the digestive tract is around 72 hours. If there are more resources required when there's inflammation, the cells may not get the support they need to repair as quickly as they should. This can lead to changes in the barrier function of the gut, meaning there is a higher risk of the intestinal contents flowing out of the gut and into the bloodstream. For example, it can make it easier for estrogens that are not yet broken down to be reabsorbed.

What happens when there's too much estrogen in circulation? You already know the answer! It causes conditions associated with estrogen dominance including endometriosis, fibroids, painful menstrual cycles and those dreaded PMS symptoms.[49]

Another area to consider is how the gut regulates cholesterol. Cholesterol, produced by the liver, is one of the compounds that forms progesterone and estrogen. If cholesterol is not eliminated or processed correctly by the gut, it can have effects on optimal hormone balance.

It's not only sex hormones that can become messed up with imbalances in the types of microorganisms that live in the gut. For one, a large amount of your happy hormone, called serotonin, is regulated by the little critters. If they are keeping a close eye on its levels, you're left at a greater risk of developing anxiety and/or depression.[50]

Optimal thyroid function can also be linked to what's happening in the gut. Those little critters that live in the digestive system are super important when it comes to ensuring that your inactive T4 hormone becomes T3. In fact, around 20 percent of the conversion rate takes place in the intestines, but it's only when you have enough of the good type of bacteria in your gut to do so. If you don't, you're losing out on a whole chunk of this process, and as you know, without enough T3, you're left with those dreadful symptoms of an underactive thyroid such as fatigue, weight gain, and even hair loss.[51] Something else to think about when it comes to thyroid function and the effect that the gut has is the absorption of nutrients. When you have poor digestive function, you're also likely missing out on getting those much-needed nutrients such as selenium, iodine, zinc and iron to the thyroid. It's plain to see that gut health is critical for thyroid health!

Estrogen Metabolism

Phase 1 Detoxification:
Happens in the Liver

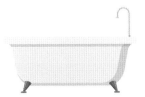

Imagine estrogen is water, filling up a bathtub. Your body uses 3 pathways to metabolize estrogen:

2-OH Estrogen:
Less carcinogenic and preferred pathway. We want to use 60-80% of this pathway.

4-OH Estrogen:
More carcinogenic and can lead to DNA damage (oxidative stress). We want to use 7.5-11% of this pathway.

16-OH Estrogen:
Can cause things to grow. We want to use 13-30% of this pathway.

Phase 2 Detoxification:
Also Happens in the Liver

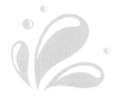

Imagine the estrogen (water) is draining out of the bathtub, is the drain slow or fast? This all depends on your COMT gene function.

Fast COMT gene function —> Better estrogen metabolism, although this can present with symptoms of its own.

Slow COMT gene function —> Estrogen struggles to get through the drain & out of the body

Phase 3 Detoxification:
Happens in the Gut

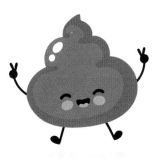

Imagine phase 3 is the sewer pipe that drains the estrogen out.

If you're dealing with gut pathogens, constipation, dehydration and more, this can cause estrogen to get reabsorbed back into the body.

Then there's insulin. Insulin is regulated by a specific lactobacillus species. If there is an imbalance in the gut microbiota, there may be subsequent problems with insulin.[52]

We already mentioned the compromise of the intestinal barrier function above, leading to leaky gut. Leaky gut has other implications in hormonal imbalances. For instance, the more we look into why women develop tissue growth outside of the uterus, which is what happens in endometriosis, we see that issues with the gut may give us additional clues. With the bigger holes in the intestinal walls, it acts like a poorly functioning filter. Instead of keeping most of the contents inside the intestine, whatever is in there has the potential to escape. In endometriosis, there is evidence to show that changes in the gut bacteria and inflammation may contribute to the development of endometriosis,[53] and while these mechanisms are still under investigation, it is an interesting angle to look at.

As you can see, addressing what is going on in the depth of your digestive system is critical to hormonal balance, and working on the body from the inside out is surely a positive way to help to settle the effects of hormonal imbalances.

The HPA-T Axis: Adrenals & Thyroid

You're going to get used to it, we promise . . . but the medical field loves acronyms! Even though you're likely going, the HPA-T *whaaaat?*, trying to remember the hypothalamic-pituitary-adrenal-thyroid axis is a mouthful!

Ok, so it is important that you know what the HPA-T axis is and what it does, and especially that it involves areas of the brain—namely the hypothalamus and the pituitary gland—and that these are interconnected with what takes place in the adrenals and the thyroid glands.

First things first: You've already been introduced to the pituitary gland, the major endocrine gland. Now comes the hypothalamus. It's a significant brain region that is responsible for keeping things in zen. Basically, its function is to maintain balance—be it weight, body temperature, breathing, blood pressure, sleep cycles, emotions, thirst, sex drive . . . you get the point, right? Everything that goes on in the body has highs and lows, but it's the job of the hypothalamus and the signals or hormones it releases and responds to that allows that zen to come back.

As you can imagine, hypothalamic dysfunction can have serious knock-on effects in many other areas of your body; just go through the list above to reiterate the gravity of the situation.

So, we mentioned hormones. Right.

The pituitary gland, a little gland in the brain no bigger than a pea, releases all kinds of chemicals that go on to signal other glands and organs to perform a specific function. In this case, the adrenal glands (situated right at the top of each kidney) and the thyroid gland (that one at the front of your neck).

When we refer to the HPA-T axis, we're really talking about a trigger, namely a stressful stimulus, that gets the hypothalamus all out of whack, which then talks to the pituitary gland to release hormones so that the adrenal and thyroid glands respond in a way that will eventually lead to a state of homeostasis.[54]

The hypothalamus activates the pituitary gland by releasing two chemicals called CRH (Corticotropin-Releasing Hormone) and TRH (Thyrotropin-Releasing Hormone).[55] The pituitary gland then responds, releasing ACTH (adrenocorticotropic hormone) and TSH (thyroid stimulating hormone). ACTH triggers the adrenal glands to release cortisol and TSH tells the thyroid to release T4. Unfortunately, T4 is not a strong hormone, so the body converts it into its most active form, which is known as T3.

With cortisol and T3 flooding the body, signals are sent back to the hypothalamus and pituitary gland to say, "Thanks, job well done, we're all good and we can return to homeostasis." Sounds great, doesn't it?

What if there's a problem? What if that stress stimulus doesn't go away? Job deadlines, bills to pay, health issues, aging parents, children that need to be in school, living through a pandemic . . . those will all contribute to a stress stimulus that doesn't turn off as it should. Now, you have constant signaling from the hypothalamus to tell the pituitary gland, adrenal glands and thyroid to keep working. Initially, this may be ok, but after a long period of time, there are just not enough resources for the adrenals or the thyroid to cope. They begin dampening their response.

We often refer to the stages of GAS (general adaptation syndrome) when this happens.[56]

The first stage is alarm. The body naturally copes with the stressor as we've described above.

Next, you enter the resistance stage, in which the body tries to recover from the initial stress but remains on high alert, just in case the threat is still there. If the stress remains, the body usually learns to cope at these new levels. Resources are still available and you may feel that you're doing well, but if you were to look at the markers such as blood pressure, cortisol levels, thyroid output etc., from your baseline to where you are now, you would notice a jump. There is also an increase in DHEA (which we discussed earlier as the precursor to your sex hormones), as it's also involved in adapting to a stressful stimulus.[57]

During this stage, you'll also be more irritable, easily frustrated and your mind will likely dart all over the place when you're trying to concentrate. You're ready to fend off danger, after all, but it never presents itself.

It's important to note that during this stage, you'll likely see a spike in the hormones being produced by the adrenal glands and the thyroid, namely T4, but you may see a decline in the TSH levels as the pituitary gland tries to help out.

On top of that, cortisol can mess with the production of the thyroid gland and, instead of converting T4 to T3, cortisol pushed T4 into reverse T3 (rT3), another inactive form of the hormone, which could then lead to an increase in TSH after a while.

Keep the stress responses going and you'll reach the last stage: exhaustion.

In this stage, the body can no longer compensate. You reach a point where you're mentally, physically and emotionally spent. This is where burnout happens. Your tolerance to stress sinks, you risk depression and anxiety, and you begin to struggle with the effects.

This is when your adrenal and thyroid glands start to show signs of decompensation. You'll likely see irregular cortisol levels when you test them, and your thyroid output may be low, and your TSH sky-high as the pituitary gland tries to compensate and maintain that now elusive homeostasis.

In order to keep up with the cortisol demands that are now tanking, the body may take essential resources that make sex hormones and convert them to cortisol instead. DHEA starts to decline,[58] as does testosterone, and you're now no longer able to make estrogen in the right amounts, which means you may lose your menstrual cycle as a result, which is known as hypothalamic amenorrhea.

Stress, whether it is physical or emotional, has a profound effect on the body and can really mess with hormonal balance, never mind all the forms of balance that are needed to maintain optimum function of your body systems. It may well be worth checking in on your stressors to determine the effect that they're having on your hormones, and in a few short pages, we'll be giving you some strategies to help you to manage those stressors so that your HPA-T axis is able to maintain that zen we all want.

Thanks, Mom & Dad: Genetics

In this section, we're talking about genes. It can get a little heavy, be warned, but stick with us and we're positive that you'll be glad you did as the level of understanding where things can go wrong will increase ten-fold.

First things first, to get the formalities out of the way: When we're talking about genes, we're really referring to the code that the body uses to perform a specific function. For example, when you start your computer, everything that you do works because there is a code running in the background, dictating what effect each action has. It's the same with the body.

Now, genes typically use proteins as messengers or signals. The gene and the enzyme may have the same name. However, the gene would be written in italics, and the enzyme it codes in standard format. For example, *TNF*, the gene that encodes TNF-alpha, is a proinflammatory gene that codes for the inflammatory molecule or cytokine that's associated with many diseases. Don't worry, you'll pick this difference up quite quickly as we go along.

Gene mutations are of critical interest in health and disease. Because a gene is put together using various components (called base pairs) that are rapidly sequenced when you are growing as a fetus, errors creep in when the base pairs are being matched for certain genes, just like typing too quickly can cause typos. Essentially, gene mutations are like typos in your genetic material. As with typos in writing, these gene typos can cause problems with the instructions they are trying to dictate.

It can be overwhelming to think about whether dirty genes are going to lead you down a path of disease. The beauty here is that genes are not your destiny. While they can have a significant impact, you have the ability to regulate them—turn them off, if you will—and allow your body to function as it should, despite your genetic tendencies.

When it comes to hormones, there are a number of genes that may either optimize, enhance, or interfere with hormone production depending on what type of typo has crept in. We'll get into those now.

COMT

COMT is one of the most significant genes when it comes to estrogen. It's the gene that codes for the proteins that help break down and clear used up estrogens during Phase 2 of detoxification in the liver so that they don't reactivate and cause trouble.[59] A well-running *COMT* pathway means that estrogens are detoxified and eliminated from the body effectively, which has significant implications not only for managing symptoms related to imbalanced estrogen levels, but also for estrogen-associated disease such as breast and ovarian cancer.

People suffering from heavy periods, PMS, fibroids and endometriosis often need to think about their *COMT*. It may be running too slowly because of a mutation, or perhaps, there is too much pressure being put on it.

You see, *COMT* function can also be slowed by exogenous estrogens. Exogenous estrogens are compounds we are exposed to in the environment that mimic the role of estrogens in the body. Things like heavy metals (think lead, cadmium, aluminum and mercury to name a few), as well as plastics, birth control pills and fire retardants, for example, can mimic estrogen. With high exposure to these xenoestrogens, the body's load increases and, with it, the risk of estrogen dominance.

Higher levels of estrogens cause a vicious cycle for *COMT*. The higher the estrogen load, the less *COMT* is able to function at an optimal level, and the higher the estrogen load becomes.

MTHFR

At first glance, you may think this is a swear word, but rest assured, it's a simple acronym for a not-so-simple gene. *MTHFR* stands for Methylenetetrahydrofolate reductase, which is a mouthful, and why we use the "cute" acronym instead.

Ok, so *MTHFR*, what does it do?

In short, *MTHFR* is the code that is responsible for producing MTHFR, the protein of the same name. *MTHFR* is essential for the way your body takes the nutrients you get from food and converts them into forms that can be used. It is responsible for methylation, or control of folate pathways, which are further involved in DNA and protein processing and repair. If *MTHFR* is not working as it should, neither will MTHFR. Poor output of MTHFR can affect hormones, neurotransmitter levels, cognitive health, your digestive health, energy balance, cholesterol levels and more.

While still a controversial topic, mutations in *MTHFR* have been implicated in PCOS.[60] Studies in this area are ongoing but, with the information we have from smaller studies, we can begin to consider how mutations in *MTHFR* can affect the condition.

There are typically two mutations in *MTHFR* that have been investigated (the C677T mutation and the A1298C mutation), but it appears that the C677T mutation is most strongly linked to an increased risk of PCOS. Further research into this association is highly anticipated.

Another way that *MTHFR* mutations can affect hormone levels is how they impact methylation. As mentioned above, methylation is the folate pathway that is primarily involved in DNA and protein repair. It gets a little more complicated. Methylation is also involved in deactivating toxins in the blood. Estrogens, while they're critical to function, become toxic if they are not dealt with in the right way after the body has used them. Methylation is important for deactivating estrogen so, if there is a mutation that causes methylation capacity to become reduced, then estrogens can become a problem, leading to estrogen dominance. There is evidence to suggest that this mechanism may play a role in the development of endometriosis, where undermethylation may impact the risk of developing the condition.[61]

We also need to look at stress and therefore, cortisol, when we speak about *MTHFR*. Mutations in this gene have been shown to enhance the perception of stress, particularly in those with C677T. With an increase in the perception of stress, there is an increase in the demand on cortisol output by the adrenal glands and a higher risk of adverse reactions relating to it.[62]

MAO

MAO codes for the enzyme called monoamine oxidase (MAO), which is responsible for breaking down the chemicals serotonin, dopamine and norepinephrine. They are neurotransmitters that are involved in feelings of pleasure, reward, aggression and the regulation of sleep.

MAO-A is commonly associated with the X chromosome (women typically have XX and men XY chromosomes) and is highly sensitive to estrogen. Estrogens dampen *MAO-A* output, which is actually a good thing, as it allows more of the happy hormones to circulate in the body. Women of reproductive age, and who have typical levels of estrogen, benefit greatly from this mood-regulating relationship, but those whose estrogens are out of whack can experience some nasty side effects. For example, at menopause, when estrogen levels plummet, *MAO-A* may begin to become more active, leaving you with a higher risk of mood imbalances as a result of lower availability of serotonin.[63] Increased *MAO-A* activity has also been implicated in the intensity of hot flashes and night sweats in women going through menopause.

Sluggish *MAO-A* function can cause levels of the neurotransmitters to rise, which can have an impact on how you behave, which as you can imagine, may lead to seriously aggressive and/or violent behaviours.[64] The phenomenon appears more often in men, as they only have one X chromosome, which means they don't have the second X chromosome to back up the *MAO-A* activity.

CYP1A2

CYP1A2 mutations have been implicated in endocrine disorders.[65] Because it's a gene that is involved in detoxification of xenobiotics (chemical substances that are foreign to the body) in the liver, poor functioning of the gene may increase the risk of toxic accumulation. The role that mutations in this gene may have on hormones is an indirect one. These chemicals may also be considered endocrine disrupting chemicals (EDCs), which alter the way the body manages hormone levels, and can include changes in androgen, estrogen, thyroid hormone and aromatase activity.[66]

BHMT

BHMT is responsible for directing the enzyme that controls the levels of the amino acid methionine. Methionine is an essential nutrient in the methylation process, so any changes in *BHMT* may have an indirect, but profound effect on hormones as a result.[67]

While it may be scary to consider all of the things that could go wrong as a result of your genes, it's important to say, once again, that your genes don't control your destiny. Yes, they may have a significant impact when activated, or turned on, but they can also be mediated, or turned off, with the right support.

I've Got the Power! The Mitochondria

There's a tiny but extremely powerful cell that you'll find in almost every other cell in your body, and it's called the mitochondria. While it's a mouthful, it plays an integral role in how your cells function. We often refer to it as the battery pack of the cell, which produces energy called ATP, allowing the cell to do what it needs to do and stay alive.

The mitochondria are also highly specialized in their role relating to hormones. They're able to not only release hormones, but produce them, too. They're involved in the manufacturing of the major precursor hormone called pregnenolone, which goes on to produce your steroid hormones, which, you guessed it, include estrogen, progesterone, androgens and cortisol in their relative tissues, like the ovaries and testes, as well as the adrenal glands.

Mitochondria are also important regulators of the thyroid hormone, where they process the hormone in the specific target tissues across the body. We also need the mitochondria for making and secreting other hormones, like insulin, which is involved in blood sugar control. Without the mitochondria, insulin release would be a mess, as would your blood sugar and your ability to use the nutrients in the food you eat as a source of energy.

On the other hand, hormones help to maintain the function of the mitochondria. So you can see why, when either the mitochondria or your hormones are out of balance,[68] things can go seriously wrong.

One of the most important sites to consider in mitochondrial dysfunction are those that are located in the adrenal glands. Here, the mitochondria are a major producer of pregnenolone, which, as mentioned above, converts into DHEA, testosterone, estrogen, progesterone and cortisol in the respective tissues.

When the adrenal glands are under duress during stressful emotional or physical periods, you can guarantee that the mitochondria are working at full capacity. They are working hard to ensure the body has enough energy to continue to function under this pressure. If this pressure continues, pregnenolone is not used to keep your sex hormones at their necessary levels. Oh, no—pregnenolone is used to keep making cortisol, that critical hormone needed to keep the body alert in the face of danger.

Keep the pressure on, and you'll start to notice. Not only in how anxious and wired you feel, but how irregular your menstrual cycle becomes. It may even disappear altogether. The body is simply saving pregnenolone for more important things, like keeping you alive.

The only way to regulate this effect is to manage the stressors. When the body is allowed to get back into a state of balance and the adrenals and their mitochondria are no longer expected to continuously ramp up due to the demands, you can expect to see the return of balance to the hormones, too.

Other Common Factors

Did you know that men and women have varying risks of viral infections? It's true.

When researchers looked into whether men or women are more prone to infection by the influenza virus, or the flu, they found that because of higher estrogens in women, particularly during their reproductive years, they have a higher degree of protection against the virus. Estrogen reduces the virus's ability to cause widespread inflammation in the body, and so even if there is infection, the symptoms may be milder.[69]

Estrogen plays a significant role in the maintenance of the immune system, which is why, when estrogens are low, for example during perimenopause and menopause, women may have more severe flu symptoms. On the other side of the spectrum, if estrogens are too high, and there is estrogen dominance, it can have the opposite effect. Instead of providing even more protection against the virus, as one would expect, because it is so anti-inflammatory, it can cause an imbalance in inflammatory and anti-inflammatory processes, which ends up causing a heightened immune response and a more severe response to the infection.

In men, testosterones offer a degree of protection against inflammation during a mild or moderate infection. If testosterone levels are not up to scratch, and there is instead a profile of estrogen dominance, for example, men will also experience a worsening of flu infections.[70]

Heavy metals are a common but often overlooked cause of hormonal imbalance.[71] Heavy metals, including lead, cadmium, mercury, copper, arsenic, nickel and aluminum, can build up to toxic levels if the body is ineffective at clearing them through detoxification (think back to the section on genes and how they can affect detoxification ability).

Mercury toxicity, for example, has been associated with PCOS, thyroid imbalances, PMS, infertility and the worsening of menopausal symptoms.[72] One of the ways mercury disrupts your sex hormones is that it may lower progesterone output, which can lead to the symptoms of high estrogen, and we know that's never a good thing.

Another consideration is that the build-up of toxic metals can physically change the adrenal glands, which alters their ability to function optimally. It's the same for the thyroid gland, and many women with thyroid issues can trace the dysfunction back to a metal toxicity. In men, research shows that occupational exposure to high levels of metals also causes testicular injury and changes in sex hormone output. There's additional evidence to show how toxic metals disrupt the ability of the pancreas to produce the right amounts of insulin, which may cause diabetes.

Exposure to mold and developing mold toxicity when the body can't effectively manage the toxins that mold releases can mess with your hormones. Women experience severe PMS, infertility, heavy periods, thyroid imbalances,[73] early menopause and night sweats, while mold toxicity in men can lead to erectile dysfunction and night sweats.

The reason? The toxins in mold, known as mycotoxins, can have direct hormone-mimicking effects, leaving the body with symptoms relating to those associated with higher-than-normal hormone levels. Mycotoxins can also have an indirect effect. Through inflammation and immune disruption, mycotoxins can cause further trouble with the endocrine system and the balance of hormones.[74]

Simply being exposed to mold and the particles being breathed in through the nose can have dramatic effects on hormones, particularly cortisol. The toxins trigger a fight-or-flight response as soon as they touch the nerves involved in smell, situated in the back of the nose, causing the body to think it is in danger. Imagine living in a moldy apartment or being exposed to mold every day you enter your place of work. There's little wonder why this chronic exposure has such a devastating effect on your hormones and your health!

With the increase in use of electronic devices, we're always interested in determining the impact they may have on health. We're not talking about stooped necks and thumb pain—we're talking hormones, of course. Electromagnetic fields (EMFs) are transmitted via radio waves. They're part of our everyday communication and are a hot topic currently. They have been shown to alter nerve impulses within our cells and may affect the output of the pituitary gland, with chronic and long term exposure.[75] As you know from previous chapters, the master endocrine gland—the pituitary gland—prompts the production and release of all of your hormones. If pituitary function is disrupted, so are all of your other hormones.

Now that you know all about what causes the rollercoaster ride that is the current state of your hormones, it's time to get into what you can do about it!

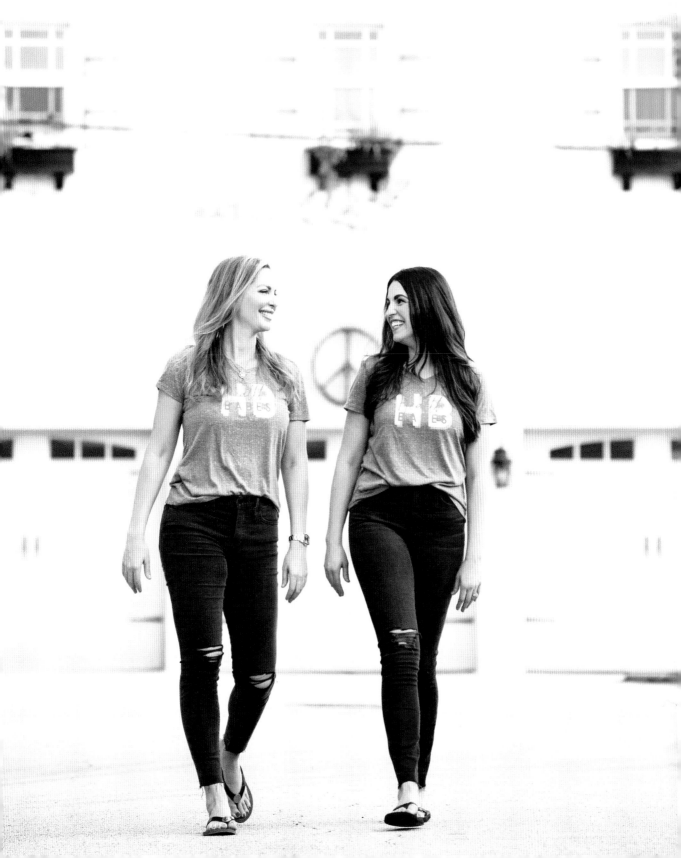

Four

GETTING DOWN TO BUSINESS, QUICK, CHEAP & EASY

There has been a *ton* of information on hormones, what they are, how they work and how they happen to lose track of what they're supposed to do.

You'll be glad to know, however, that the steps to correcting them and giving them a nudge in the right direction are not as laborious or tough to do. So, breathe, relax, and let's get you fixed up, shall we?

Eating Better, Not Less

Many of you may have thought it was a hormonal issue that has led to changes in your weight, but without the right information in your toolkit, you may have started to restrict your eating as a means to balance it out. After all, everything you read online says you need to eat in a calorie deficit to lose weight, right? And the food tracking app that you're so diligently using says you should be eating around 1,200 calories, right?

Wrong. And *wrong*!

Eating in a calorie deficit, when the deficit is too high, can cause weight *gain*. Eating 1,200 calories is what a toddler should consume each day! Enough said.

Now, it may terrify you to think that you actually have to eat more to lose weight, and you may wonder what kind of hocus pocus science this really is, but hear us out . . . Think back to *all* of the wonderful information you have just read. What was the one theme running through the entire book so far?

Did I hear you say, "balance?" Excellent!

And yes, we need balance not only to maintain a healthy weight, but to support our hormones, and every body system in general. If you're not eating enough, you're out of balance. When you don't have enough nutrients in your system, your body feels like it's under threat, and what happens when your body feels threatened? Your hormones suffer. Everything is at risk of shifting out of balance.

In fact, when you're not eating enough, your body will start to produce more hunger hormones. It's a survival mechanism, a reaction to stress,[76] and its aim is to prevent starvation. It happens without you even realizing it. All of a sudden, you become ravenous. You just want to eat, and you want to eat *now.*[77]

It's not likely that you go for the big green salad or bowl of vegetables when you're that hungry. Instead, it's highly likely that you go for and over-consume the high calorie, refined foods. It leads to a vicious cycle of binging and restricting, which has further effects on your weight and your hormones because of the inflammation it can cause.

There's also the implications that restrictive eating has on other aspects of your health. As you get older, your bones are already losing minerals and increasing your risk of osteoporosis as a result of lowered estrogens. Add to that poor nutrient intake, and the risk of osteoporosis increases.[78]

Your metabolism also suffers, as do your energy levels. Again, all of these imbalances can simply be corrected if you eat enough of the right types of foods.

The bottom line is that food is there to nourish your body and give it the resources it needs to function. We have an entire section about what to eat, what to avoid, how to eat and when coming up in a bit, so stay tuned!

If Pooping Is Wrong, I Don't Want to be Right

No one likes toilet talk, but we have to say, it's something you need to get used to. Your bowel habits tell you a lot about your health, and believe it or not, what goes into the toilet has a critical role in hormonal balance.

Getting comfortable with taking note of how often you go, when in the day you go and what comes out is not only helpful for figuring out what may be going on, but can be critical for taking the steps that are right for you and your body.

So, let's talk poop for a minute, and we'll start with constipation.

If you were to guess the difference in the risk of constipation in men versus women, what would you say? Don't know?

Well, according to the British Medical Journal,[79] women are twice as likely to suffer from constipation as men, and you can probably guess why: estrogen.

Not only does estrogen slow down the transit time of food through your digestive tract, leading to constipation, but constipation itself can cause estrogen levels to soar, which causes a worsening of the problem. You see, there are estrogen receptors found all throughout the lining of the digestive tract. If there is more estrogen in circulation, as is the case with estrogen dominance, these receptors are all too happy to latch onto available estrogen, which causes muscle contractions to reduce in frequency. If the muscles aren't contracting very often, there's a slowed propulsion of food towards the rectum, and that leads to constipation and the inability to feel fully cleared out even when you do manage to go.[80]

The trouble with constipation is that the waste that the body is trying to get rid of is now staying put, where it doesn't belong. We've already spoken about the gut microbiota at length in Chapter 3 (page 39), but it's important to touch on it again now. The critters packed inside the colon only know one thing: They get to work fermenting and processing whenever there is a substance in their reach. This time, unfortunately, it's old waste that has already been fermented and processed, but they can't differentiate, so they believe that they need to re-ferment and reprocess the waste.

It becomes a bit of a mess, really, with more gas being produced and the development of a swollen and gassy belly.

On top of that, there are species of bacteria that produce a compound called beta-glucuronidase, which reactivates used-up estrogens that have been set for elimination. When the estrogens are reactivated, they can be reabsorbed back into circulation, causing higher levels of estrogen, but they can also attach to those receptors in the digestive tract, further impeding transit and movement.[81]

Another area to consider is what constipation does to the levels of inflammation in the digestive tract. Chronic digestive inflammation can upset the barrier function, leading to a condition we call leaky gut syndrome.[82] Basically, without a proper barrier, the permeability of the gut increases, which means that the contents within the digestive tract are more easily able to flow through into the bloodstream. The implications here aren't great. Larger undigested food particles, bacteria, viruses and yeasts, as well as toxins and estrogens, can get into the blood, where they don't belong. And you've already learned that toxins can lead to hormonal imbalance, and that excess estrogens flowing around in the body can cause a lot of trouble.

It also affects progesterone. Chronic inflammation, especially at the gut level, can cause progesterone receptors to stop working as they should. Your body may continue producing enough progesterone, but with the desensitization of the receptors, the messages aren't getting through, and you can suffer the fate of low progesterone symptoms such as weight gain, irritability, insomnia, infertility, headaches and low libido.

Don't forget your thyroid hormones.[83] Recall that a large deal of the conversion of the inactive T4 to the active T3 happens in your gut. An unhappy, inflamed and leaky gut leads to an unhappy conversion of the thyroid hormones, and you may struggle with low thyroid issues, despite being on medication. We also can't forget about the effects an unhappy gut can have on stress and the production of the hormone cortisol. Inflammation = cortisol, as simple as that.

It doesn't stop there . . .

Insulin resistance is yet another risk of leaky gut syndrome due to inflammation and poor utilization of nutrients, as are sleep and mood disorders, as the hormones melatonin and serotonin are made in the gut.

Essentially, what we're saying is that in order to maintain overall hormonal balance, you need to poop. Regularly.

To do so, you need to support the gut environment with lots of good quality fiber, drink your water, consider taking probiotics if indicated—or better yet, eat fermented foods, and give your gut lots of love with good, clean food. It's an essential piece of the puzzle for hormonal balance and one that we'll be referring back to when we talk about the food choices for hormonal health.

If you're doing everything listed above and still not seeing improvements, you may need to work with a functional medicine practitioner and do thorough testing on the gut to see exactly what is going on. We do this with all of our patients.

Show Your Middle Child More Love: The Liver

Giving your liver some love is key to optimizing your hormone balance. From what you've already read, you're well aware of the role of the liver in its detoxification capacity, which means it has a role in processing and eliminating hormones that have been used up by the body.

The detoxification process is an interesting one. How well it functions is critical to whether your hormones behave, or whether they become unruly.

In order to fully understand the liver's role here, we need to consider the ins and outs of detoxification. We also need to understand *why* detoxification is important.

Detoxification is performed in two phases. The first phase, conveniently called Phase 1, is simply put, the process of taking a potential toxin and turning it into something harmless.[84] Phase 1 uses nutrients such as B vitamins, amino acids, vitamin C, zinc, vitamin A and flavonoids and it processes compounds through processes known as oxidation, reduction, hydration, dehalogenation and hydrolysis.

As a result of these processes, toxins are rendered harmless, but there's a catch: free radicals are formed. You must have heard of free radicals before. Those nasty, unstable compounds that can have potentially devastating effects on your tissues and cells? Because of that, we want to neutralize them as quickly as possible, and we do so by making sure we have enough antioxidants available. Antioxidants are extremely helpful here. They bind to the unruly free radicals, calming them down and rendering them harmless. They are the perfect match.

Too many free radicals and/or an insufficient supply of antioxidants is a recipe for disaster. Not only do free radicals cause inflammation, but they can also damage the liver tissues itself, interfering with its detoxification capabilities. It's for this reason that we need to show our liver a lot of love by providing it with an abundance of the nutrients it needs to function, lots of rich antioxidants and trying to lessen the load of toxins it needs to process.

Next is Phase 2. It's a little more complex and involves the process of conjugation. During this phase, another compound is added to the toxin, transforming it into a molecule that is easily mixed with water. This way, it becomes a cinch to get rid of it, along with other forms of waste, in the urine and stool. Nutrition becomes even more important during this phase. No longer is your liver using simple vitamins and minerals, so now it needs something more "hardcore." Proteins are the name of the game and, more specifically, sulfur-containing products of protein breakdown, namely the amino acids called cysteine, methionine and taurine.[85]

When Phase 2 detoxification is sluggish, your body doesn't take it well. We see a myriad of symptoms starting to show, such as joint pain and swelling, headaches, digestive disorders, immune issues and autoimmune conditions developing, intolerance to chemicals, asthma and, you guessed it, hormonal issues.

The next question to answer is why detoxification is important or, should we say, why you need to keep thinking about your liver and the hard work it puts in every second of every day. If that's on your mind, you're more likely to take action to support it, and let's be honest, it will take all the support it can get. Of course, the liver and your other detox organs like the kidneys, colon, lungs and skin are all crazy good at what they do. The trouble is that for many of you—and the reason you're reading this book in the first place—is that something is not right. Your liver is probably *not* the get-up-and-go liver of the past, and it *does* need some pure, undivided TLC.

Why? You, me and everyone else live in a toxic environment. Look around you. There's plastic, tap water, pesticides, processed foods, metal, chemicals and pollutants at every turn. You may not even be aware of half of the chemicals and/or toxins that your body is processing—here's looking at you lifting, anti-aging, moisturizing, SPF-containing day creams. You put these onto your face every day, and while they may feel amazing, your liver is screaming, "No more!" Added to that, as a society, we're eating out more frequently, drinking more coffee and alcohol, and generally putting more toxins into our bodies than we even know exist.

Most of these affect the complex second phase of detoxification, which means it backs up. The liver doesn't just throw in the towel, shrivel up and stop working—it deals with the problem, and the easiest way to cope? Your liver allows some of the other compounds in the body to re-enter into circulation, and yes, that includes half-metabolized hormones[86] that have already been through Phase 1. Guess which one is going to wreak havoc on your already stressed hormonal system—estrogen, which gets recirculated and therefore contributes to overall estrogen load.

How do you know if you need to spend some good quality time with your liver? Here are some of the top factors to look out for:

- Intolerance to alcohol
- Intolerance to coffee
- Swelling of the feet
- Bad breath
- Heartburn
- Reacting strongly to heavy chemical smells (perfume, paints, bleach etc.)
- Strong body odor
- Dark urine or stool
- Struggling to lose weight
- High cholesterol
- Hormonal issues (sleep issues, brain fog, irregular or heavy periods, mood swings etc.)
- Blood sugar imbalances
- Skin breakouts or rashes
- Digestive issues

Many of these are general symptoms that can explain a lot of different conditions, but maybe looking into the health of your liver can help to resolve some of them.

Supporting the liver is easy. Food is critical, and we'll talk about that in the next chapter, but you can also be more mindful of the toxins you're exposed to on a daily basis. Try to stay away from processed and packaged foods as much as possible and try to buy organic food, or at least wash your fruit and vegetables well before storage and preparation, drink filtered water, and opt for natural personal hygiene and home cleaning products where possible. Every little bit helps, and your liver will certainly love you back for it!

The Three S's: Sex, Stress and Sleep

It's time for the next step in the journey to a renewed sense of health and well-being, and there's no better way to start that off than to talk about sex . . .

"O" MY!

Sex isn't all about pleasure. Oh, don't get us wrong, the pleasure part of it is pretty darn amazing, but there are so many more incredible reasons to keep going back for more. For one, all of that movement sends blood and nutrients rushing through your body. Of course, this is good for the health of your heart, your brain and other organs, but it's also *great* for your vagina! Without sex, there's little need to send valuable resources down south, and it can contribute to vaginal dryness and other less favorable symptoms many of you would likely attribute to getting older.[87]

Reaching orgasm is also a great way to lower stress and that critical stress hormone cortisol,[88] more of which we'll talk about in a bit. It's basically nature's Prozac and Xanax all rolled into one![89] Think about the sense of happy calm you feel after an orgasm. The climax of it all sends happy hormones (endorphins) and bonding hormones (oxytocin) flowing through your brain. It's also the reason you feel sleepy after sex; the body, simply put, is in a state of sheer bliss and not even the thought of a work deadline the next day can take that away.

The best thing about orgasm is you don't have to rely on a single person to get there. We have to start letting go of the traditional ideology that you need a partner to have sex or reach orgasm. There are more than enough hardworking people out there developing technology that allows us to climax on our own. Now that you know how important it is, there's more than enough reason to give it a try. This is all about you and your health, and I can assure you, it's far better than chocolate.

Signs of Sluggish Liver Function

INTOLERANCE TO ALCOHOL

INTOLERANCE TO COFFEE

SWELLING OF THE FEET

BAD BREATH

HEARTBURN

REACTING STRONGLY TO HEAVY CHEMICAL SMELLS (PARFUME, PAINTS, BLEACH ETC.)

STRONG BODY ODOR

DARK URINE OR STOOL

STRUGGLING TO LOSE WEIGHT

HIGH CHOLESTEROL

HORMONAL ISSUES (SLEEP ISSUES, BRAIN FOG, IRREGULAR OR HEAVY PERIODS, MOOD SWINGS ETC.)

BLOOD SUGAR IMBALANCES

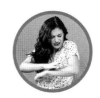

SKIN BREAKOUTS OR RASHES

DIGESTIVE ISSUES

ALWAYS SEEK SERENITY

We cannot say this enough, but stress management is likely one of the most essential tools you can master when it comes to regulating your hormones. As you've come to realize, stress has such a profound effect on every aspect of your health, and chronic exposure to the hormones related to the stress response is going to leave you feeling less than healthy and happy.

There are so many ways that you can tackle stress head on, each and every day. It's all about ensuring that you're putting your parasympathetic nervous system first. It is, after all, the system that is responsible for your rest and digestive state, and it's impossible to support your hormones if you're always in fight or flight mode.

Let's talk about the vagus nerve for a minute. It's the main sensory nerve that runs along the back side of the body and is essentially the functional part of the parasympathetic nervous system. With every stress-management technique you put in place, you're supporting the vagus nerve, and in doing so, you're also allowing your parasympathetic nervous system to work.

While relaxation, such as taking time to meditate and quiet your body and mind, can work wonders, there are additional ways to support the vagus nerve. Humming, gargling, chanting and singing, for example, cause vibrations to stimulate the vagus nerve. If you're more into the extreme, you can experiment with cold water, too. It might sound counterintuitive, but the shock of cold water on your body can have a contrasting supportive action on your vagus nerve. Splashing your face with cold water, going out into the cold with minimal clothing for a few seconds, or turning the shower onto its coldest setting for a few seconds are all easy ways to experiment with cold stimulation of the vagal pathways.

Exercise is another great way to support vagal tone. Exercise itself can stimulate a stress response, but here's the thing . . . It's an *adaptive* stress response, which helps the body become generally more resilient to stress, i.e., the body is better at balancing the rest and digestive system with the fight-or-flight system.

Stress management may seem time-consuming and complicated. It doesn't have to be. If you only have 5 minutes a day, you can still practice active stress management, which can have really great overall benefits by reducing the output of cortisol and the effects it has on the body.

What can you do in 5 minutes? Breathe.

Breathing is one of the easiest, cheapest and most effective ways to manage stress.[90] Did you know that shallow breathing is one of the hallmarks of stress? In order to combat it, you simply have to focus on breathing deeply. Each day, practice taking long breaths in through the nose, trying to fill not only your lungs, but your belly too, then slowly releasing it through the mouth. Five to eight cycles is all you need to allow the body to get into a natural state of calm. Once you have the hang of doing this morning and night, you can start using it as a technique to cope with in-the-moment-stress. At even the slightest feeling of discomfort, stop what you're doing and breathe . . . simple, yet effective.

If you have the time and resources to do so, you can incorporate more intensive stress management techniques into your daily routine. Take a longer break to meditate and breathe. Incorporate gentle exercises into your day, get out into nature or do something fun. You can even seek professional help, for example, through counseling or cognitive behavioral therapy. All of these are really great ways to manage stress.[91]

IT'S ALL ABOUT THE ZZZZZ'S

Without sleep, you cannot function. Without sleep, your health becomes a rapidly growing snowball, wreaking havoc as it careens down the side of a steep mountain face. If that sounds dramatic, then we've made our point.

Sleep is, after all, a timeout that the body takes to repair itself.[92] If these careful repair processes are not completed on a routine basis, things are going to break. Cortisol levels soar, insulin becomes dysfunctional, the thyroid takes a hit, weight management becomes difficult (if not impossible), toxins become tough to manage, and that snowball grows and grows and grows.

We get it, it's tough to prioritize sleep. Between work, family, the great shows they have on Netflix and the trouble we have sleeping anyway (hot flashes, hello!), we'd be surprised if there were very many of you reading this book who shrugged their shoulders and said, well actually, my sleep is ok!

So, what do we do about it? One, sleep needs to be prioritized. Set a time that you want to go to sleep every night, and no matter what, don't deviate. Also, think about the environment you sleep in. Is it inviting for sleep? Is it a place you feel at peace?

Make sure your bedroom is cool, but not too cold, dark enough to keep you asleep even if there is light outside, and that it is quiet. If you need to use earplugs and/or an eye mask, do it! You can thank us later when you wake up feeling refreshed, happy and ready to put a spring in your step.

Forget about the fountain of youth. Sleep is the elixir of life and all that is good.

Five

USING DIET TO SUPPORT YOUR HORMONES

What you put on your plate can either make or break your hormones. Now, remember we don't want to starve ourselves, or for that matter, restrict ourselves to the point we can no longer continue and end up giving up, binging on foods that we know aren't helping.

We want to nourish our bodies, and still derive some pleasure from eating!

What to Eat

The very first thing we need to note is that this is a whole-food, nutrient-dense diet. It means that we make every effort to give our bodies the building blocks it needs to support the function of every body system,[93] including those responsible for hormone balance. It is also meant to reduce inflammation, a significant cause of imbalances and hormone disruptions.[94]

The second key concept is that you need to eat enough. It's the only way your body is going to get the nutrients it needs to function and keep you satiated and feeling good about what's on your plate.

FRUITS AND VEGETABLES

Have you ever heard that you should fill half your plate with vegetables at each meal? This is not a myth. Along with the health benefits of the vitamins, minerals, polyphenols, flavonoids and antioxidants you get from eating colorful vegetables, you're bound to feel full and satisfied as a result of the fiber they contain—oh, and healthier bowel movements, too.

In addition, a specific type of vegetables, called cruciferous vegetables, contain nutrients that support the liver detoxification pathways, those essential pathways that help to detox your hormones. Go for all of the colors of the rainbow, but be sure to include broccoli, kale, arugula, cabbage, cauliflower, Brussels sprouts, bok choy and collard greens into your everyday hormone balancing diet.

Fruit is a great way to satisfy cravings and add more healthy nutrients to your diet. Choose low glycemic index fruit such as berries for up to two servings a day. Limit those sweeter tropical fruits to a small portion on occasion. Fruit can affect blood sugar, and thus insulin levels, if they are eaten in bigger and more frequent portions. Look at fruit as a functional part of the diet, whereas restriction is important for overall health.

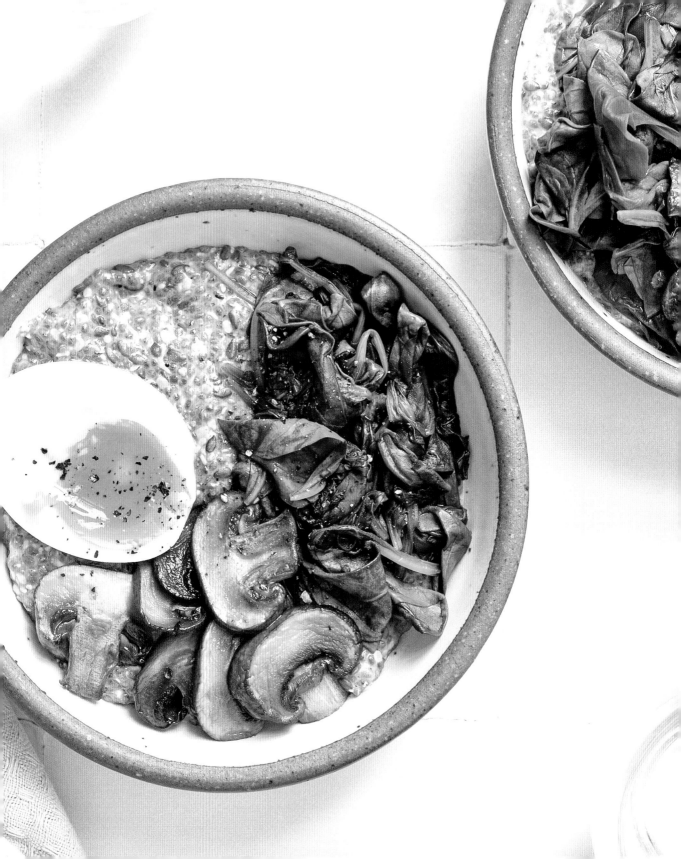

PROTEINS

Proteins are a must-have in any diet. They include amino acids, which are the building blocks of your lean mass, they contribute to satiety at meals and, of course, they play a role in hormone production.

Animal proteins, such as grass-fed and grass-finished beef, organic chicken, wild caught fish, organic turkey, lamb and pork, as well as eggs, are included in a hormone-balancing diet. Protein powders made from hydrolyzed beef, bone broth and collagen may also be included for an alternative and convenient source of protein. Be sure to check the ingredients here! Avoid anything with unrecognizable ingredients, ingredients you can't pronounce and/or anything artificial.

FATS

Besides the delightful texture and flavor fat can bring to a meal, fat has an important role in the body. It is used to build the membranes of most of our cells and plays an essential part in the health of the nervous system. Fats also have a role in hormone regulation. These little globules build other compounds that have hormone-like functions which, in turn, affect the endocrine system.[95]

That's why including fat in your diet is critical—healthy fat, that is.

Healthy fats come from sources that are animal- and plant-based. Think grass-fed butter, ghee, tallow and lard. Plant-based fats should include nuts, seeds, their oils and butters, as well as avocado, olives and their oils.

Additional sources of fat in the diet will come from the fatty fish you eat—for example, salmon, mackerel and tuna, as well as from egg yolks and the fat you'll get from eating meat.

CARBOHYDRATES

We all love carbohydrates, and yes, they can—and should—be included in a healthy diet! Unprocessed, complex carbohydrates, that is.

Cassava, plantains, sweet and regular potatoes, yams, squash, peas, rutabaga and parsnips are all a great source of nutritionally dense carbohydrates you can eat.

Don't forget to add lots of fresh and dried natural herbs and spices to your meals. They're full of flavor and all have their very own health properties to contribute.

MACROS

Unfortunately, there is not a one-size-fits-all formula for this. This is very independent of each person, depending on what your hormones are doing. The good news is that our bodies are very good at telling us what they like. If you notice that higher carbohydrates in your diet make you feel sluggish and bloated, then you will probably do better on a moderate to low carb diet.

On the other hand, if you notice that you start eating a lower-carb diet and your hair falls out and you're lethargic, then you may need to add more healthy carbs to your daily meals.

What to Avoid

One of the most important aspects of eating nutrient dense is to reduce inflammation. There are six main culprits in our diet that cause inflammation, and we really want to encourage you to stay away from them as much as possible.

1. SUGAR

Sugar is a big no-no for hormones. While you know that refined sugar is the worst of the offenders, any form of sugar in high amounts can cause as much of a problem, even those that are marketed as being healthy like coconut sugar, honey and maple syrup. While these forms of sugar are better than processed sugar, they should only be consumed in moderation. Those with PCOS may consider completely eliminating them.

Unfortunately, they all do the same thing: spike your blood sugar and place a higher demand on insulin.[96] High insulin levels in turn affect SHBG, which means estrogen is less likely to be deactivated and excreted from the body. Do you remember the section on estrogen dominance? It's just not worth it. Instead, if there's a real need for something sweet, include small amounts of fruit into your diet, or consider using natural sweeteners such as stevia or monk fruit sweetener on occasion. Cinnamon and pure vanilla extract can also give the illusion of sweetness in foods, so use these liberally.

2. DAIRY

Dairy can be an issue for some and not others. Dairy can have a lot of beneficial nutrients if tolerated. All dairy contains various amounts of hormones including estrogen and progesterone. Milk derived from a pregnant animal will contain significantly higher levels of hormones compared to that which you'll get from a nursing cow. It's hard to tell what is what when you're selecting your milk at the grocery store. Having hormonal imbalances means that this additional source of hormones can be quite bothersome. Think about your skin. If you struggle with breakouts, you may be having a negative response to dairy.[97]

Dairy is also notoriously hard to digest in some individuals, causing rapid and significant digestive upset. If you've ever had milk and had to rush to the restroom soon afterwards, this could be why.

If you find you do not do well with dairy, some dairy milk alternatives include coconut milk or almond milk. Just make sure they come from good sources and are not filled with a lot of fillers like gums. The fewer ingredients, the better. You can also make your own if you're feeling frisky.

3. GRAINS & LEGUMES

Speaking of sugar, grains are carbohydrates that are converted into sugar through digestion. It's not only the sugar component that we are worried about when it comes to grains; it's also their affect on inflammation.

Many of you may be substituting animal protein in your diet with beans and lentils. Of course, we agree that more plant materials in the diet are amazing, but . . . we want to watch our intake! Why? Both grains and legumes contain a couple of compounds we call anti-nutrients; that doesn't sound like a good thing, does it? Well, no, it's not.

The first of two that we need to mention is phytic acid. It's a compound that these plants contain to protect themselves. It's not great for you, as it can reduce the absorption of iron, zinc and calcium—three essential minerals you need not only for overall health, but hormonal health, too.

The biggest trouble is for those of you who eat mostly a plant-based diet, as these minerals are likely available in smaller amounts in any case, and there is a higher risk of mineral deficiencies as a result.

The next compound to consider is lectins. Lectins pass through the digestive system undigested and can cause inflammatory conditions in the gut to worsen.

These anti-nutrients really detract from the health aspect that grains and legumes may provide, so it's best to avoid them or only eat them in smaller amounts if you do enjoy them.

If you do decide to have these, make sure you are properly soaking and preparing them before eating. Soaking them for at least 4 hours (prior to cooking) and cooking them in an Instant Pot® can help reduce phytic acid.

4. INDUSTRIAL SEED OILS

Now that you know which fats are good for you, we definitely need to clarify the fats that aren't. Anything that has been overly processed needs to be stopped right at the door, and that means all processed seed oils.

These oils are highly inflammatory, which means they have significant consequences on your health. There is evidence that they can lead to infertility and gut issues, some of the factors you likely now know a lot more about when it comes to your hormones.

The main offenders in industrial oils are sunflower seed, soybean, corn, rapeseed (canola), safflower and cottonseed oils. The reason they are like poison to the body is that they are heated to extremely high temperatures, processed with harmful chemicals such as petroleum-based solvents and then deodorized. It sounds as awful as you think! These oils are chemicals, and are doing nothing good for you or your health, so stay away. Instead, use olive, coconut or avocado oil.

5. ALCOHOL

Some whole food nutrient-dense food plans will include the allowance of a small amount of alcohol. While you're going to make your own decision on whether to include it or not, we've listed it under the foods to avoid to make sure you know how to navigate alcohol if you do decide to include it.

Although it has been said that there are some health benefits of drinking a small amount of red wine, alcohol is a toxin, and it must be viewed as such, especially when we look at everything we've addressed regarding liver health and the detoxification of hormones. The second point is that alcohol may contain grains and sugar, two of the no-nos listed above. If you're to include alcohol, do so in moderation and opt for organic dry wines, vodka (stay away from those that are made from grain), gin and tequila.

List #1 The Health Babes' Food List

VEGETABLES

- Artichokes
- Arugula
- Asparagus
- Bamboo shoots
- Beets
- Bell pepper
- Bok choy
- Broccoli
- Brussels sprouts
- Cabbage
- Carrots
- Cauliflower
- Celery
- Collard greens
- Cucumber
- Eggplant
- Endive
- Fennel
- Garlic
- Green beans
- Kale
- Kimchi
- Leeks
- Lettuce
  (all varieties)
- Mushrooms
- Mustard greens
- Okra
- Onions
- Peppers
- Pumpkin
- Radishes
- Seaweed
- Sauerkraut
- Spinach
- Squash
- Sweet potato
- Tomatoes
- Turnips
- Zucchini

DRINKS

- All Teas
- Bone Broth
- Coffee
  (organic is best)
- Club Soda
- Lemon Juice
- Lime Juice

FLOURS

- Almond flour
- Coconut flour
- Psyllium husk
- Other nut flours

SWEETENERS

- Monk Fruit
- Stevia

MEATS
(Grass-fed is best)

- Bacon
  (nitrate &
  gluten free)
- Beef
- Beef Jerky
  (nitrate &
  gluten free)
- Bison
- Chicken
- Duck
- Lamb
- Organ meats
- Pork
- Poultry
- Steak
- Turkey
- Veal
- Venison

FRUITS

- Apples
- Avocado
- Bananas
- Berries
- Blueberries
- Cantaloupe
- Cherries
- Coconut
- Cranberries
- Goji berries
- Grapefruit
- Grapes
- Kiwi
- Lemon
- Lime
- Mango
- Olives
- Orange
- Papaya
- Pear
- Pineapple
- Plum
- Pomagranate
- Raspberries
- Rhubarb
- Strawberries

NUTS & SEEDS
(Soaked is best)

- Almonds
- Brazil nuts
  (good for selenium,
  thyroid)
- Chia seeds
- Flaxseed
- Hazelnuts
- Hemp seeds
- Macadamia
- Pumpkin seeds
- Pecans
- Pine nuts
- Sesame seeds
- Sunflower seeds
- Walnuts

FISH & SHELLFISH
(Choose wild and fresh
when possible)

- Cod
- Crab
- Halibut
- Lobster
- Mackerel
- Mussels
- Oysters
- Salmon
- Sardines
- Scallops
- Shrimp
- Trout
- Tuna

CONDIMENTS

- Apple Cider Vinegar
- Balsamic Vinegar (gluten free)
- Coconut Aminos
- Cocoa Powder
- Dill Pickles (no preservatives
  or coloring added)
- Dried Herbs & Spices
- Fish Sauce
- Horseradish
- Hot Sauces
- Mayonnaise
  (paleo)
- Mustard
- Salsa
- Tabasco Sauce
- Vinegars
  (gluten free)

STARCHES

- Beets
- Cassava
- Jicama
- Konjac shirataki
  noodles
- Plantains
- Pumpkin
- Rutabaga
- Squash:
  acorn,
  butternut,
  spaghetti
- Sweet
  potatoes
- Taro
- Turnips
- White
  potatoes
- Yam
- Yucca

FATS

- Avocado oil
- Beef tallow
- Butter (grass-fed)
- Coconut butter
- Coconut oil
- Duck fat
- Extra Virgin
  Olive Oil
- Ghee (grass-fed)
- Lard
- Macadamia oil
- Mayonnaise (paleo)
- MCT Oil
- Olive Oil

OTHER

- Eggs
  (pasture-raised)

List #2 Eat in Moderation

- **Processed meat.** Sausage, bacon and jerky. Make sure they are gluten, sugar and soy free. Organic / free-range meat is preferable.

- **Whole fruit.** Approximately 1-3 servings per day, depending on your blood sugar balance. Favor low sugar fruits like berries and peaches over tropical fruits, like apples and pears.

- **Nuts and seeds.** A maximum of a handful per day, preferably soaked overnight and dehydrated or roasted at low temperature (150 degrees) to improve digestibility. Favor nuts lower in omega-6, like hazelnuts and macadamias, and minimize nuts high in omega-6, like brazil nuts and almonds.

- **Green beans, sugar peas and snap peas.** Though technically legumes, they are usually well tolerated.

- **Coffee and black tea.** Black, or with coconut milk. Only if you don't suffer from fatigue, insomnia or hypoglycemia, and only before 12:00 PM. Limit to one cup (not one triple espresso, one cup).

- **Dark chocolate.** 70% or higher in small amounts (i.e. about the size of a silver dollar per serving) is permitted.

- **Vinegar.** Apple cider vinegar is especially well tolerated.

- **Restaurant food.** The main problem with eating out is that restaurants cook with industrial seed oils, which wreak havoc on the body and cause serious inflammation. You don't need to become a cave dweller, but it's best to limit eating out as much as possible during this initial period.

List #3 Foods to Avoid

· **Dairy.** Some people do well with raw dairy and even some conventional dairy, like cottage cheese and heavy cream. We believe dairy, in all forms, should be tested to see how you respond and eaten in moderation if tolerated.

· **Grains.** Including bread, rice, cereal, oats, or any gluten-free pseudo grains like sorghum, teff, quinoa, amaranth, buckwheat, etc.

· **Legumes.** Including beans of all kinds (soy, black, kidney, pinto, etc.), peas, lentils and peanuts.

· **Concentrated sweeteners, real or artificial.** Including sugar, high-fructose corn syrup, maple syrup, honey, agave, brown rice syrup, Splenda, Equal, Nutrasweet, xylitol, etc. (*Stevia is a good alternative).

· **Processed or refined foods.** As a general rule, if it comes in a bag or a box, don't eat it. This also includes highly processed "health foods" like protein powder, energy bars, dairy-free creamers, etc.

· **Industrial seed oils.** Soybean, corn, safflower, sunflower, cottonseed, canola, etc. Read labels – seed oils are in almost all processed, packaged and refined foods (which you should be mostly avoiding anyway).

· **Sodas and diet sodas.** All forms. Alcohol in any form.

· **Processed sauces and seasonings.** Soy sauce, tamari, and other processed seasonings and sauces (which often have sugar, soy, gluten or all of the above).

How Often Should I Eat?

Are you a grazer? A meal skipper? Or someone who only eats when they're truly ravenous? Believe it or not, your eating schedule can play a big role in hormone regulation, and it can be as important as *what* you eat when it comes to balance. For each of you, this might look slightly different, and it depends on what your hormones are doing.

Those of you with cortisol or thyroid issues are better off eating regular meals. Skipping meals or fasting for too long can increase the stress effects on the body and result in further dysregulation of these critical hormones. Fasting can still help with weight management, but it is not recommended to go longer than 14 hours without food. Additionally, if you fall into either or both of these two categories, it's better for you to have something to eat within an hour or two of waking, and to rather close the kitchen earlier in the evening to ensure a 12- to 14-hour overnight fast.[98]

In those with PCOS and insulin regulation issues, intermittent fasting can be really beneficial. Going without food for an extended overnight period can drastically improve endocrine function and prevent the potential devastating side effects that chronically high insulin may have.[99] Research has suggested that a 16:8 fasting to feeding window, which means you fast for 16 hours and eat only in an 8-hour timeframe, can have significant and positive outcomes for cycle regulation, reducing body fat, regulating hormones, lowering insulin levels and managing inflammation.[100] With that being said, bio-individuality plays a big role in diet. Not all cases of PCOS are driven by insulin resistance. When PCOS is driven by adrenal gland dysfunction, for example, intermittent fasting may not be the right option. If you find yourself feeling exhausted with fasting, this may be a sign that it is not right for you.

Research also suggests the meal timing we stick to when we do eat is important. For example, grazing on snacks throughout the day may not only interfere with insulin levels, but result in a higher caloric intake than we realize, as well as put more pressure on the digestive system to work. If you're already struggling with insulin imbalances, weight management issues and less than optimal digestions, eating three meals and one snack across a 12-hour period may be helpful, which for most, would mean eating every 3 to 4 hours.

If you're not sure about when to eat, the easiest is to go with a 12-hour overnight fast and then have a meal or snack every 3 to 4 hours after that. Adjustments can be made further along the line, once your body gets used to eating nutritious, healthy foods.

Shifting Your Mindset on Your New Lifestyle

You'd be surprised how easy it is to implement healthy food choices into your day-to-day lifestyle. Losing weight and managing your hormone health is about giving food a new perspective. Instead of focusing on what you can't eat, always look at what you can eat. In the end, eating to balance your hormones doesn't mean you can't enjoy food. Just wait until you see the delicious foods you can make. Coming up in the next section we've got some amazing recipes to share, including a bunch of delectable desserts!

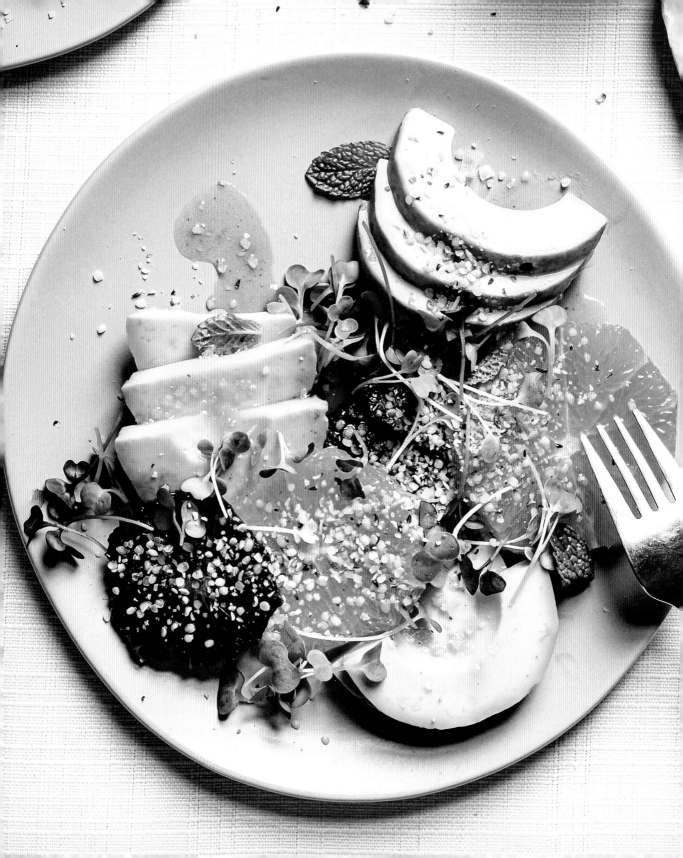

Six
HORMONE-HEALTHY RECIPES

Let food be thy medicine. This quote is very true when it comes to supporting hormone health. Getting in balanced meals of protein, fat, carbohydrates and fiber is essential for balanced hormone levels.

To support hormones like progesterone, testosterone, estrogen, cortisol, insulin, leptin and thyroid hormones, we need to feed our bodies a good balance of macro and micronutrients. The meals below are filled with color and will provide you with many vitamins, minerals and macronutrients to ensure your hormones are getting the support they need.

It's important to note that when you eat your meals, make sure you sit down in a non-stressful state with no distractions. We should not be eating when we are stressed or on the go. This is terrible for digestion. Digestion helps us absorb the nutrition from the foods we eat. Make sure you chew your food thoroughly. Digestion starts in the mouth. Take this time to yourself and give yourself permission to be still while you eat. Your body will love you for this.

Now that we are talking about implementing the delicious recipes below, we also need to discuss intermittent fasting.

If you incorporate intermittent fasting (IF), and are a cycling female, make sure you do this in the follicular phase of the menstrual cycle. This is days 1 through 14 in an average 28-day cycle. Your body can handle fasting better in this phase because we have fewer hormonal fluctuations. Your body is a little more sensitive in the luteal phase and tends to do better when you are getting in more meals. This is very important to note with people who are also perimenopausal. Our hormones are extra sensitive, so the timing with IF is

important. People in menopause tend to handle fasting well because they have fewer hormonal fluctuations.

Men tend to handle fasting better than women. If you are a man and reading this, just make sure you feel good while fasting and listen to your body. If you feel lethargic and have low energy, fasting may not be right for you. If it gives you energy and mental clarity, you need to listen to that. You can also play around with fasting windows.

We recommend that you start with a simple 12-hour fast and then you can go up to a 16-hour fast if desired. This means that you do not eat for the allotted time and eat two to three meals in the eating window.

If you are not fasting, make sure you start your first meal (breakfast) within an hour of getting up. Your breakfast should be a balance of protein (about 1 gram of protein per pound of body weight), fat and fiber. This is important for blood sugar optimization, which is important to start your day off right. The good news is all of our meals focus on getting balanced micro and macronutrients.

For lunch, we provided a lot of hearty salads filled with color, along with soups that are easy for leftovers. Eat this meal in the middle of the day after giving your digestion a break after breakfast. Dinner should be treated the same as lunch. Give your digestion some time to rest after lunch and enjoy one of the amazing dinner options listed under Dinner. This break will also help stabilize your blood sugar.

We hope you love these meals as much as we love them! See you in the kitchen!

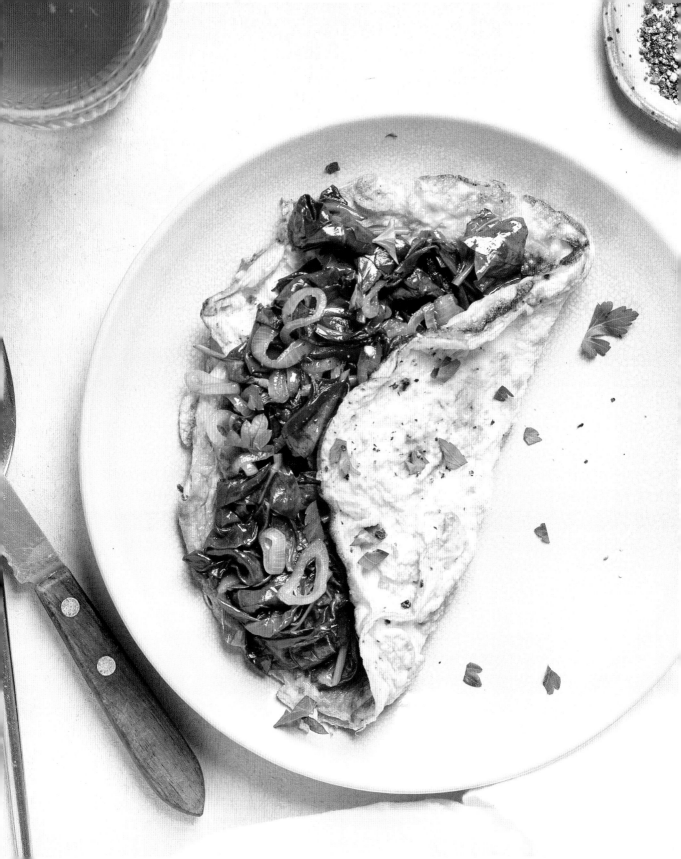

BREAKFASTS

SPINACH & SHALLOT OMELET

Yield: 2 servings

Need a quick and easy weekday meal? Give this omelet a try. Not only a breakfast meal, an omelet also provides healthy sources of protein and fat, guaranteed to keep your tummy full until lunch. Here we suggest adding spinach, but you can chop and add any other vegetables you have on hand. This omelet is easy, healthy and satisfying, something we can all get behind!

1 tbsp (15 ml) olive oil

1 shallot, sliced

1 clove garlic, minced

2 cups (60 g) spinach

4 eggs

Salt and pepper

1 tbsp (14 g) grass-fed butter

Heat an 8-inch (20-cm) skillet over medium heat. Add the olive oil and then the shallot. Cook the shallot for 3 to 5 minutes until it is tender and then add the garlic. Cook for an additional minute and then, working in batches, add the spinach and toss with the shallots until the spinach is wilted. Transfer the spinach to a plate and then return the skillet to the heat.

Allow the skillet to heat back up for a minute or two while whisking the eggs with a pinch of salt and pepper. When the skillet is warm, add the butter. Wait for the butter to melt and then pour the eggs in. Allow the eggs to cook undisturbed for 1 to 2 minutes, and then gently lift the edges with a rubber spatula and tilt the pan so that the liquid egg mixture on top can run beneath. Do this for a couple of minutes until the top of the omelet still appears shiny and wet but there isn't enough liquid to run off. Then, carefully flip the omelet in the pan, add the spinach and shallots to one side of the egg, and fold the other side over.

Remove the omelet from the pan and serve hot.

BREAKFAST TACOS

Yield: 2 servings

Breakfast can be the most important meal of the day, and what better way to set yourself up for success than with a healthy meal that contains all of the nutrients you need, including protein, fat and carbohydrates? With these breakfast tacos, not only will your taste buds be satisfied, but you'll manage your blood sugar levels, cortisol levels and stimulate those feel-good hormones at the start of your day.

4 strips nitrate-free bacon, diced

1 tbsp (15 ml) olive oil or grass-fed butter

3 eggs, scrambled

4 medium-sized Paleo tortillas

¼ cup (45 g) cherry tomatoes, diced

2 tbsp (6 g) scallions, sliced

¼ of a jalapeno, thinly sliced (optional)

Parsley, for garnish

Heat a medium-sized skillet over medium heat. Add the diced bacon and cook, stirring occasionally, for 5 to 7 minutes or until the bacon is well browned and crisp. Use a slotted spoon to transfer the bacon to a paper towel–lined plate. Set the bacon aside, carefully dispose of the bacon grease, and then wipe the pan.

Return the skillet to medium-low heat and allow it to heat up before adding the olive oil or grass-fed butter. Swirl to coat the bottom of the pan and then add the eggs and cook, stirring frequently until the eggs are fully cooked through.

Gently heat the tortillas in a toaster oven or a clean skillet and then build the tacos by dividing the eggs, bacon, tomatoes, scallions and jalapeno amongst the tortillas. Serve garnished with parsley.

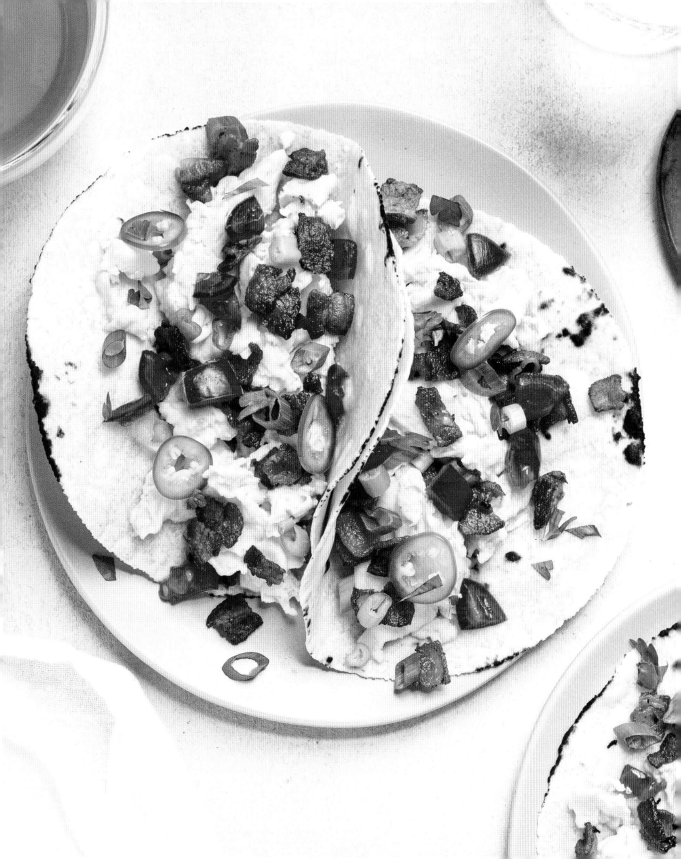

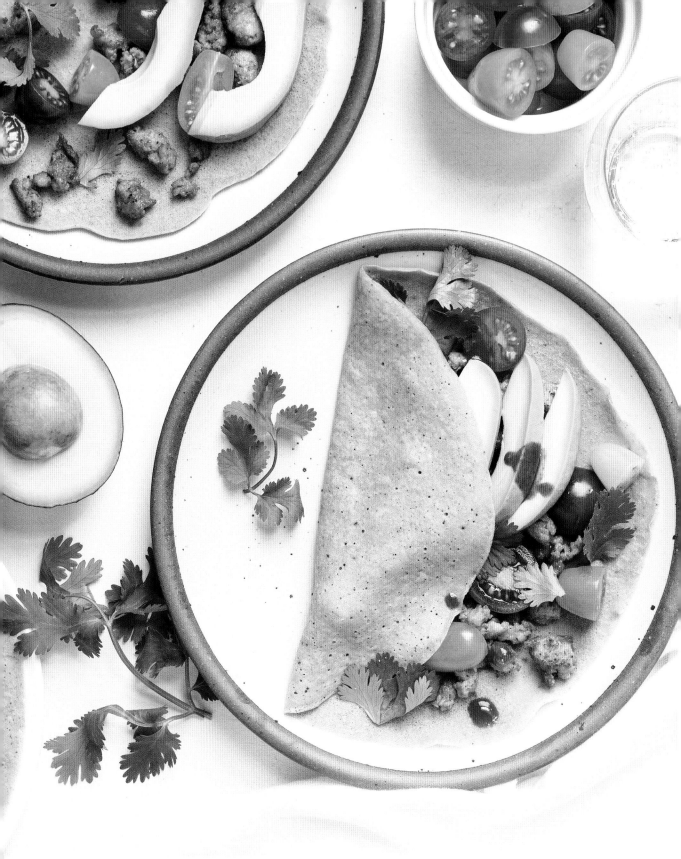

SWISS CHARD CREPES

Yield: 8 crepes

Forget green eggs and ham! Here you have green crepes and sausage. Using Swiss chard, you're not only boosting the nutrient profile of the crepes (and making them green, of course), you're adding a whole whack of fiber to reduce the blood sugar soaring effect you would typically associate with this type of meal. Keep them savory with the addition of sausage and avocado, and add a little spice, if you dare!

FOR THE CREPES

1 egg

1 packed cup (36 g) Swiss chard

½ cup (64 g) almond flour

½ cup (75 g) cassava or tapioca flour

1 tsp baking powder

¾ cup (180 ml) almond milk

¼ tsp cumin

1 tsp salt

¼ tsp pepper

Olive oil cooking spray

FOR THE FILLING

½ pound (226 g) Italian sausage

1–2 avocados, sliced

½ cup (75 g) cherry tomatoes, halved

½ cup (8 g) cilantro leaves

Hot sauce (optional)

In a blender, place the egg, Swiss chard, almond flour, cassava flour, baking powder, almond milk, cumin, salt and pepper, and then process on high speed until the batter is smooth. Heat a large nonstick skillet over medium-low heat. Spray the pan with olive oil cooking spray and then pour ¼ cup of the batter into the center of the skillet and immediately swirl it around to create a thin circle approximately 8 inches (20 cm) in diameter. Let the crepe cook for 1 to 2 minutes until the edges are set and the center no longer looks wet. Gently lift the edges all the way around with a spatula and then flip the crepe. Cook for an additional minute and then transfer the crepe to a parchment-lined baking tray or a plate. Continue this process until all the batter has been used.

Once finished, return the skillet to stove and increase the heat to medium. Remove the sausage from the casing and break it into pieces into the skillet. Cook the sausage until it is well browned, breaking it into crumbles with a spatula as you go.

To serve, place a crepe on each plate and top it with the sausage crumbles, a few slices of avocado, a handful of cherry tomatoes, cilantro and hot sauce, if using. Leftover crepes can be stored in the freezer between pieces of parchment for a month.

BROCCOLI FRITTATA

Yield: 1 (6-inch [15-cm]) frittata

Broccoli gets a bad rap for being bland or, in some cases, too bitter. It is, however, an essential item on your grocery list if you want to manage your hormones. It supports the liver in its detoxification processes, so be sure to incorporate broccoli into your daily diet. A tasty and convenient way to do that is to make these delicious broccoli frittatas.

1 tbsp (15 ml) olive oil

1½ cups (135 g) broccoli, florets and stems cut into ½-inch (1.3-cm) pieces

8 eggs

⅓ cup (80 ml) almond or other nondairy milk

1 tsp salt

¼ tsp pepper

⅓ cup (80 g) goat cheese

¼ cup (10 g) parsley or basil, for garnish

Preheat the oven to 425° (218°C), and then heat a 6-inch (15-cm) cast iron skillet over medium heat. Coat the base of the skillet with the olive oil and then sauté the broccoli until it is tender, about 5 minutes.

Meanwhile, whisk together the eggs, almond milk, salt and pepper. Pour the egg mixture over the broccoli and then crumble the goat cheese evenly over the eggs. Transfer the skillet to the oven and bake until the entire frittata has puffed and the center is no longer jiggly, for 17 to 20 minutes.

Garnish with fresh herbs such as parsley or basil.

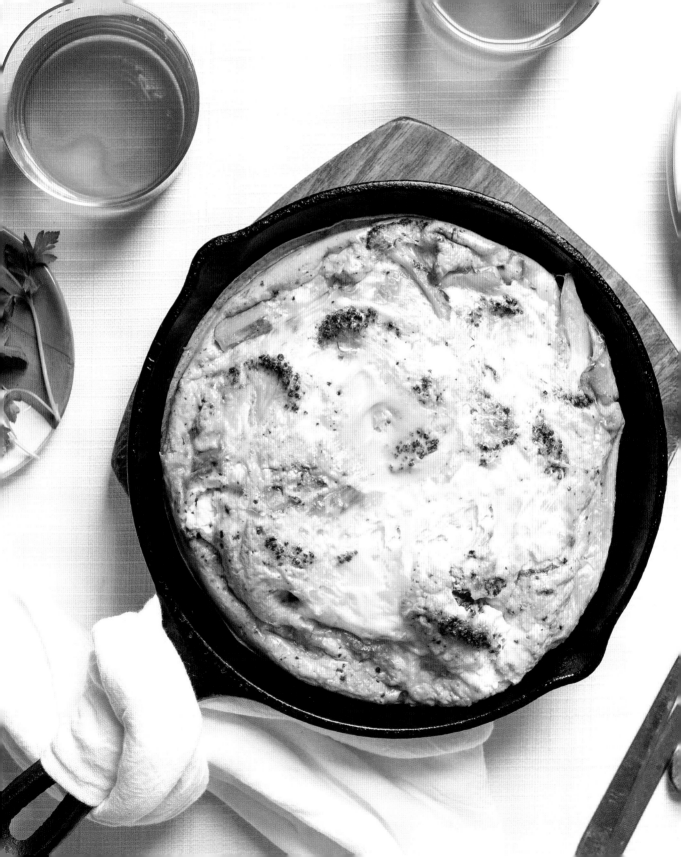

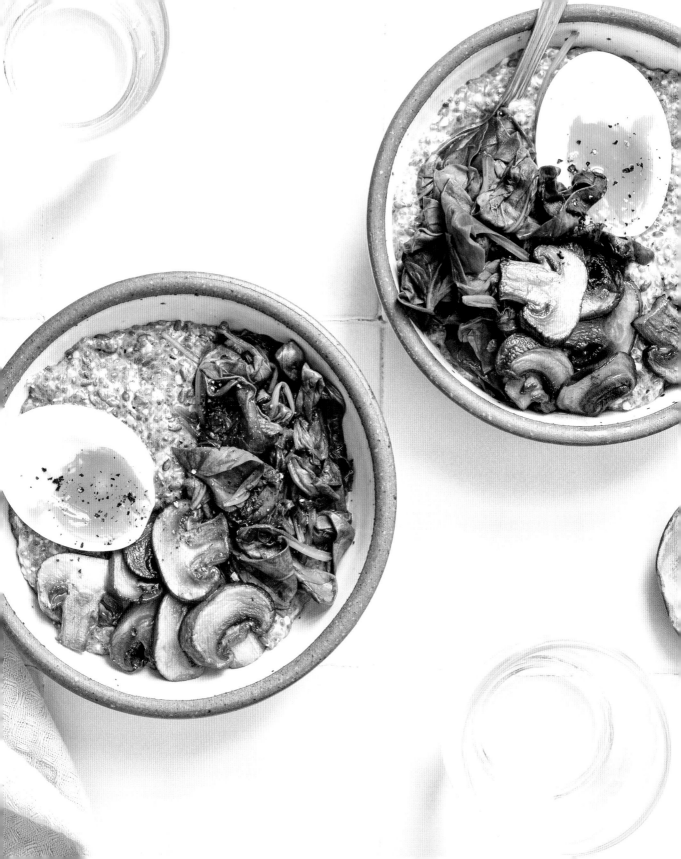

SAVORY SEED PORRIDGE

Yield: 2 servings

Here's a porridge dish that is just as good for breakfast, lunch or dinner. That's right! You can eat porridge at any meal, as long as it's this savory seed porridge! Packed with the health benefits of hemp and flax seeds, as well as turmeric, ginger, spinach and mushrooms, this is one big bowl full of goodness you can really get behind.

2 eggs

¼ cup (41 g) chia seeds

2 tbsp (20 g) flax seeds

2 tbsp (20 g) hemp seeds

⅓ cup (80 ml) coconut milk

½ cup (120 ml) water

½ tsp turmeric

½ tsp ground ginger

¼ tsp salt, plus a pinch

¼ tsp pepper

1 tbsp (15 ml) olive oil

1 cup (70 g) mushrooms, sliced

1 cup (30 g) spinach

Fill a medium-sized saucepan with water and bring it to a boil. Gently add the eggs to the water and boil for 7 to 8 minutes (for a soft yolk) and then drain the pan and run the eggs under cold water to stop the cooking process. Set them aside while you prepare the porridge.

Place the chia seeds, flax seeds and hemp seeds into a small saucepan, along with the coconut milk, water, turmeric, ginger, ¼ teaspoon of salt and pepper. Bring the mixture to a simmer and cook for 3 minutes and then turn off the heat and allow it to sit while you prepare the vegetables.

Heat a medium-sized skillet over medium heat and add the olive oil. Add the mushrooms to the pan, along with a pinch of salt, and cook until tender. Transfer the mushrooms to a separate plate and then add the spinach to the pan and cook for 1 to 2 minutes, until it is just wilted.

At this point, check on the porridge. If it has become too thick, add water 1 tablespoon (15 ml) at a time until you reach the desired consistency. Divide the porridge between bowls and then top it with the mushrooms and spinach. Peel the eggs and add them to the bowls.

EGG BITES

Yield: 12 egg bites

Don't let the stress of waking up early to make breakfast get you down! Make these easy, yet tasty egg bites in advance so you can grab and munch on-the-go every morning. Containing a rich source of nutrients and protein in the eggs and a little bit of fat from the bacon, you're guaranteed to keep your blood sugar and insulin in check with this breakfast option.

Olive oil cooking spray

5 slices bacon, diced

¼ red onion, diced

½ cup (90 g) cherry or grape tomatoes, diced

1 clove garlic, minced

¼ cup (10 g) basil leaves, roughly chopped

11 eggs

⅓ cup (80 ml) nondairy milk

1 tsp salt

¼ tsp pepper

Preheat the oven to 350°F (177°C) and spray a muffin pan with olive oil cooking spray.

Heat a skillet over medium heat and cook the bacon for 5 to 7 minutes, until crisp. Transfer the bacon to a paper towel–lined plate to drain the oil.

Toss the bacon, onion, tomatoes, garlic and basil into a bowl and then divide the mixture between the 12 muffin cups.

In a large bowl, whisk together the eggs, nondairy milk, salt and pepper. Pour the mixture into the muffin tins, filling each muffin tin to three-quarters full.

Place the egg bites into the oven and cook them for 18 to 20 minutes or until they have puffed considerably and are no longer jiggly in the center.

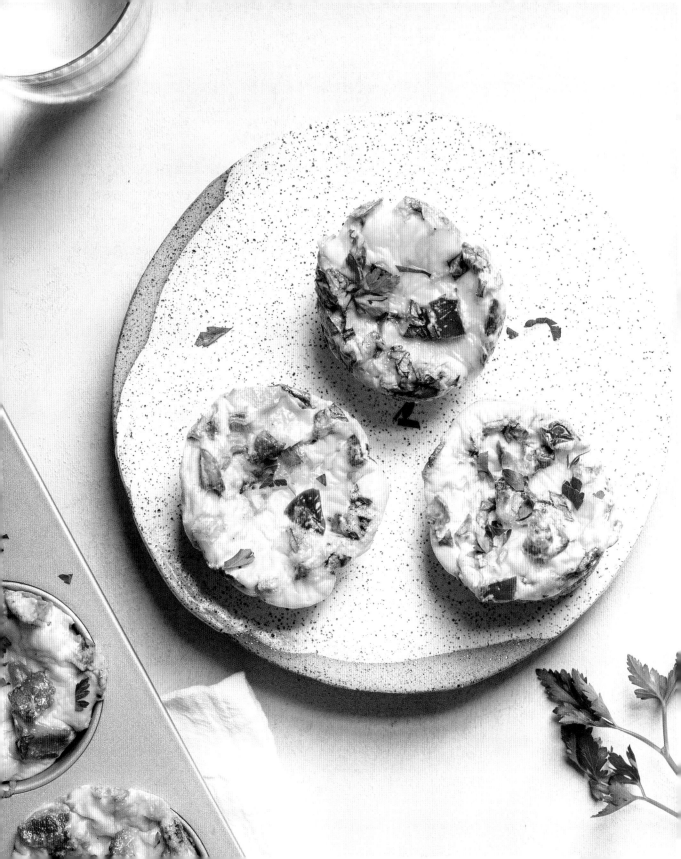

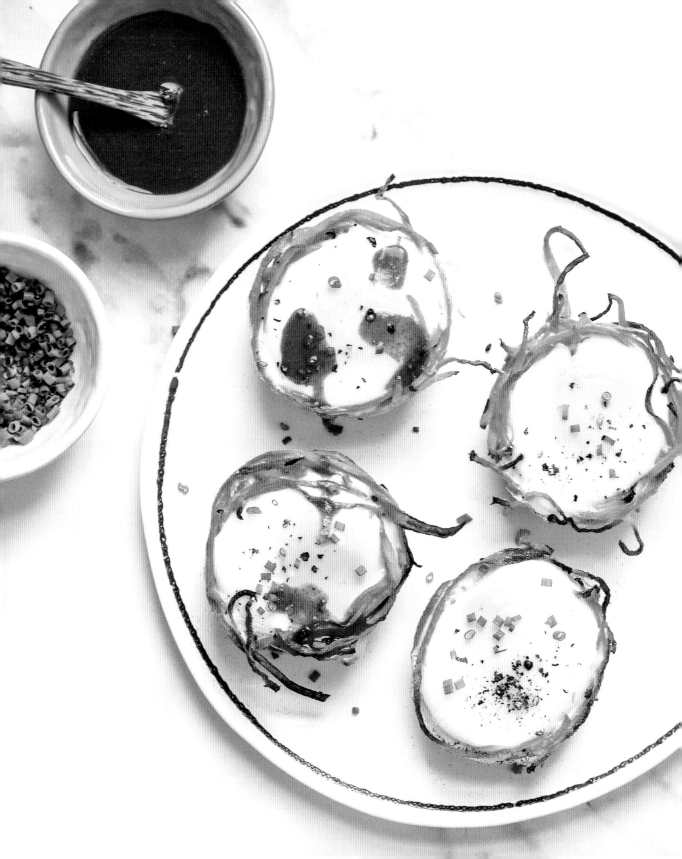

SWEET POTATO HASHBROWN CUPS

Yield: 12 servings

It's time to get a little bit fancy with these hashbrown egg cups. Don't let the name deter you—they're so quick and easy to make, and you can whip up a ton in advance and freeze them for quick on-the-go meals in days to come. While we like them with fiber- and vitamin C–packed sweet potatoes, which also have a progesterone-moderating effect, they're just as tasty with butternut squash. The protein and fat in the eggs help to balance out the little bit of starch, and you can eat them on their own with a little bit of hot sauce or add them to a side of sautéed vegetables for a heartier meal.

1 lb (454 g) sweet potatoes or butternut squash, spiralized or julienned

2 tbsp (30 ml) olive oil

½ tsp salt

½ tsp pepper

1 tsp garlic powder

Pinch of red pepper flakes (optional)

Olive oil cooking spray

12 eggs

2 tbsp (6 g) chives, for garnish

Hot sauce (optional)

Preheat the oven to 350°F (177°C). In a medium-sized bowl, toss the sweet potatoes with the olive oil, salt, pepper, garlic powder and pepper flakes, if using. Lightly spray a muffin pan with olive oil cooking spray and then divide the sweet potato mixture into the cups. Press the sweet potato down into the muffin cup and up against the side. These will shrink as they cook, so it's ok if there is a little overhang.

Cook the sweet potato cups for 10 minutes, and then remove them and use a spoon to reform the center hole if necessary. Crack an egg into each sweet potato cup and return the pan to the oven for 12 to 14 minutes or until the eggs have set but still have a little jiggle in the yolk.

Remove them from the oven and garnish the sweet potato hashbrown cups with chives and hot sauce, if desired.

HUEVOS RANCHEROS

Yield: 2 servings

If you love Tex-Mex, you can certainly work it into your hormone-healthy eating plan. Instead of loads of unhealthy ingredients, we've put a simple spin on a much-loved tortilla dish. Switch out regular tortillas for those made of coconut or other low-carb ingredients, and there's no reason to give up on your favorite foods while working on your health.

½ lb (226 g) sausage, removed from the casing

½ tsp cumin

1 tbsp (15 ml) olive oil

2 eggs

2 medium-sized Paleo tortillas

½ avocado, sliced

⅓ cup (87 g) salsa (no sugar added)

Cilantro, for garnish

Heat a skillet over medium heat and cook the sausage with the cumin until the sausage is well browned, breaking it apart with a spatula as it cooks. Transfer the sausage to a bowl, carefully wipe the skillet clean, and then return the skillet to the heat. Add the olive oil and allow it to heat up before cracking one egg into the skillet. Fry the egg, gently lifting the edges and swirling the oil around the pan until the whites are fully set and the yolk is cooked to your liking. Transfer the egg to a plate and repeat with the other egg.

Meanwhile, gently warm the tortillas in a toaster oven or a clean skillet and place onto two plates. Top each tortilla with the sausage, egg, sliced avocado and salsa. Garnish your huevos rancheros with cilantro.

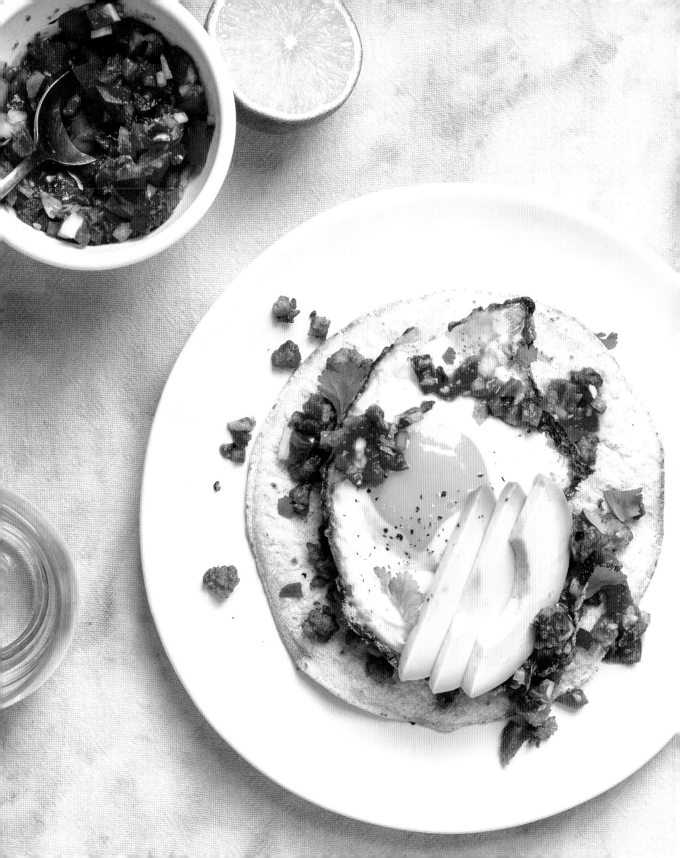

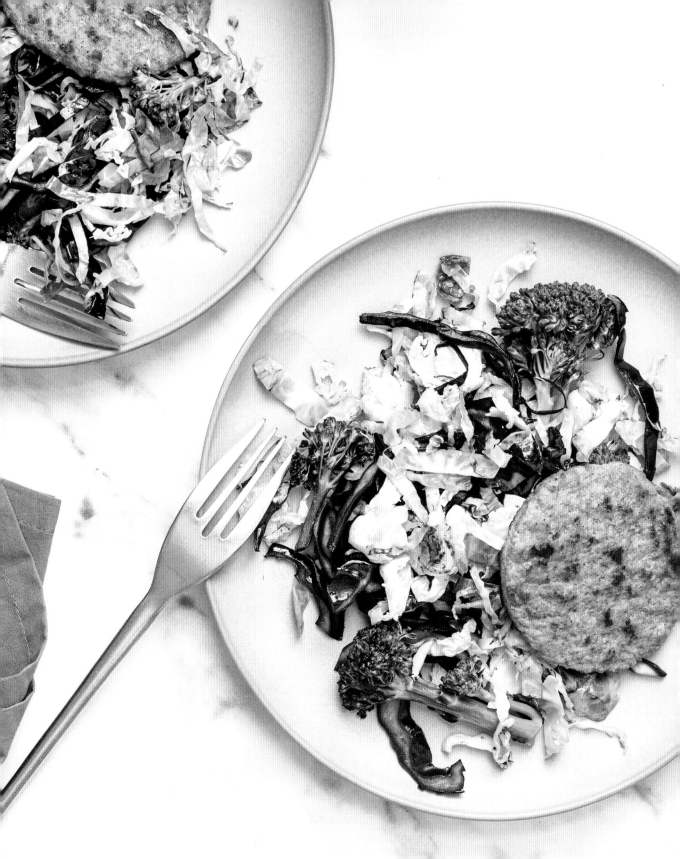

CHICKEN PATTIES WITH BROCCOLI & CABBAGE

Yield: 2 servings

Broccoli, Brussels sprouts and cabbage all fall under the category of brassica vegetables. You've learned about brassicas in this book already, but a quick recap is that they supply a sulfur source that supports the liver detoxification pathways. The liver is the most important organ for hormone detoxification, which is why these vegetables should be a staple in your diet. They're also a great source of vitamins C, A, E and K, as well as the minerals folate, calcium, iron, potassium and phosphorus. This is a meal with both health and flavor.

1 tsp garlic powder

1 tsp onion powder

2 tsp (4 g) cumin

1 tsp sea salt or Himalayan salt

½ lb (226 g) ground chicken

2 tbsp (30 ml) olive oil, bacon fat or grass-fed butter, divided

1 cup (91 g) broccoli florets

1 cup (70 g) shredded red cabbage

1 cup (113 g) shredded Brussels sprouts

In a small bowl, mix together the garlic powder, onion powder, cumin and salt.

Place the ground chicken in a medium-sized bowl and season it with one-fourth of the spice mix. Then, divide the meat into two patties. Heat a medium-sized skillet over medium-high heat. Drizzle 1 tablespoon (15 ml) of olive oil into the pan and then place the chicken patties into the skillet and cook them over medium heat until well browned, 2 to 3 minutes per side.

Meanwhile, heat a large skillet over medium heat and pour in the remaining tablespoon (15 ml) of olive oil. Add the broccoli florets, shredded red cabbage and shredded Brussels sprouts to the skillet, along with the remaining spice mix, and cook until they are tender and lightly browned, for about 10 minutes.

Serve by first placing the cooked veggies on your plate. Add the chicken patties on top and enjoy!

Note: Homemade chicken patties can be replaced with Applegate frozen patties. Use two frozen patties per serving.

POTATO PANCAKES

Yield: 6 pancakes

Years of misinformation has left many of us thinking that potatoes are a no-no when it comes to healthy eating. We say not so! Potatoes are a great source of prebiotic starch, a complex form of carbohydrates that help you to feel fuller for longer and feed your gut bacteria at the same time. Now, you can eat a small amount of regular potatoes in your weekly meals, or you can bring a five-star feel to your breakfast, lunch or dinner plate with these easy-to-rustle-up potato pancakes. We guarantee this is a dish the whole family will love.

2 lbs (908 g) russet or Yukon gold potatoes, peeled

1 yellow onion

1 egg, plus more if desired

1 clove garlic, minced

2 tsp (12 g) salt

½ tsp pepper

¼ cup (37 g) cassava flour

1 tsp baking soda

2–3 tbsp (30–45 ml) coconut oil, plus more if needed

3 tbsp (9 g) chives

Grate the potatoes and onion using the largest holes of a box grater. Squeeze out the excess water with your hands or a clean dish towel and place them in a colander to drain while you prepare the remaining ingredients.

In a large bowl, whisk the egg and minced garlic together and season them with the salt and pepper. Add the drained potato and onion mixture to the egg and toss everything well to combine. Stir in the cassava flour and baking soda until they are well combined. Divide the mixture into six patties (each should be a heaping ¼ cup [60 g]) and place them on a piece of parchment.

Heat a cast iron skillet over medium heat and then add the coconut oil. Once the oil is hot, cook the potato pancakes for 4 to 6 minutes per side until they are deeply golden brown. Work in batches to avoid crowding the pan and add more oil if necessary. Remove the patties from the pan and place them on a paper towel–lined plate.

Serve with chives and fried eggs (optional).

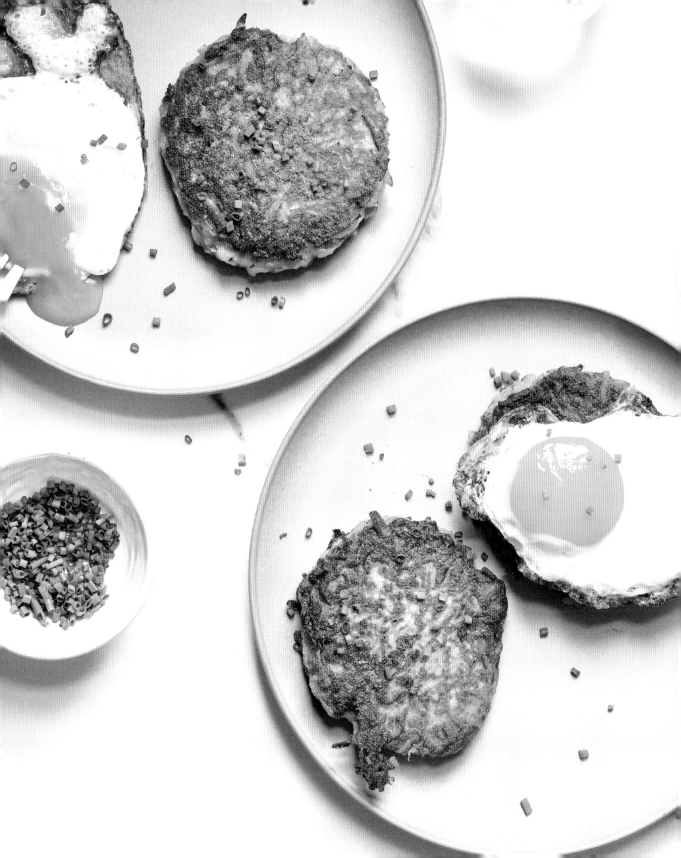

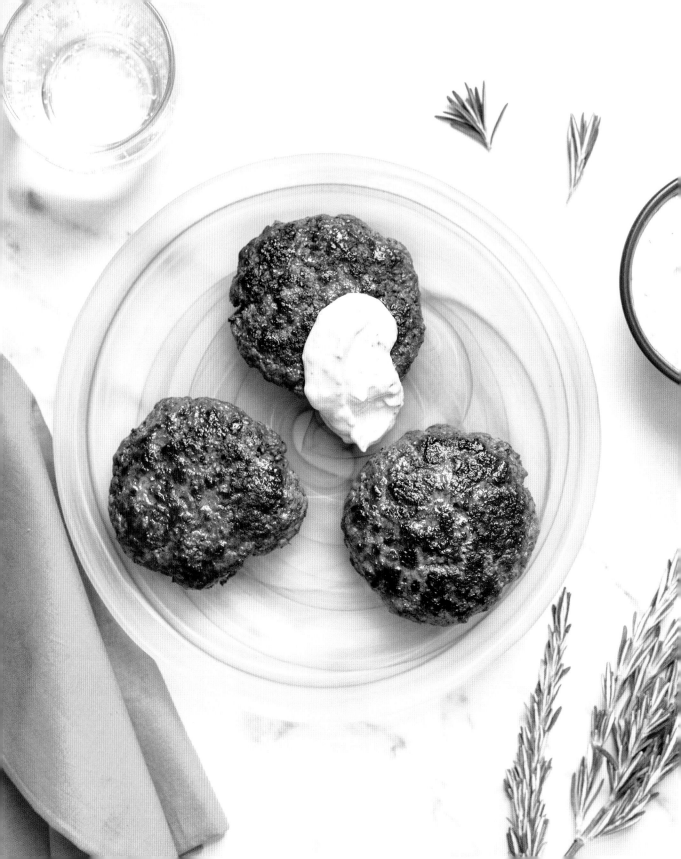

LUNCHES

BISON PATTIES WITH ROSEMARY AIOLI

Yield: 4 servings

Not only is bison a super lean source of red meat, but it's also a rich source of major minerals like iron, selenium and zinc. It's also a great way to top up your vitamin B levels. Ground bison makes tasty burgers and can be a delicious meal that can be a staple in your diet. Add this delicious rosemary aioli and you're left with mouth-watering flavor in addition to the anti-inflammatory properties of garlic and the immune-supporting benefits of rosemary.

FOR THE PALEO-STYLE MAYONNAISE (MAKES 1 CUP (240 ML))

1 cup (240 ml) extra light tasting olive oil

1 egg

Juice of ½ lemon

1 tbsp (15 ml) sugar-free Dijon mustard (we use Annie's Organic)

¼ tsp pink Himalayan sea salt

FOR THE AIOLI

1 tbsp (14 g) garlic paste

1 tbsp (2 g) minced rosemary

1 tsp lemon juice

Salt and pepper, to taste

FOR THE BISON PATTIES

1 lb (454 g) ground bison

1 tsp salt

½ tsp ground pepper

½ tsp onion powder

1 tsp garlic powder

1 tsp paprika

1 tbsp (15 ml) olive oil

First, make the mayonnaise by adding the olive oil to a canning-style jar, followed by the egg, lemon juice, mustard and salt. Use an immersion blender on low to blend the mixture until a mayonnaise-like consistency forms. Set half of it aside and place any leftovers in the refrigerator.

To make the aioli, mix together ½ cup (120 ml) of the Paleo-style mayonnaise, garlic paste, minced rosemary and lemon juice in a small bowl. Taste and adjust the salt and pepper as needed. Set the aioli aside.

In a medium-sized bowl, combine the ground bison with the salt, pepper, onion powder, garlic powder and paprika and mix well. Divide and form four equally-sized patties. Heat a large skillet over medium-high heat. Drizzle with the olive oil and then cook the bison patties for 3 to 4 minutes per side. Serve the bison patties with the aioli for a nutritiously dense lunch.

CREAMY BROCCOLI SOUP

Yield: 4 servings

If you're finding it hard to eat your daily serving of broccoli without it being smothered in loads of butter and cheese, here's an easy work-around: creamy broccoli soup. It's not only easy to make but also ensures you get all of the benefits from broccoli's liver-supporting components.

2 tbsp (30 ml) olive oil

1 onion, diced

2 celery ribs, diced

2 carrots, diced

Salt and pepper

2 chicken breasts

6 cups (1.4 L) chicken stock

2 small or 1 large head of broccoli (approximately 6 cups [546 g])

½ teaspoon turmeric

¾ cup (180 ml) almond milk or other nondairy milk

Place a soup pot over medium heat and, once hot, add the olive oil. Sauté the onion, celery and carrot with a pinch of salt and pepper until just tender, for 3 to 5 minutes. Add the chicken breasts and stock along with the broccoli to the pot. Bring everything to a simmer and then cook for 12 to 15 minutes, until the chicken is cooked through. Transfer the chicken breasts to a plate and allow them to cool slightly before shredding.

Reserve a few florets of broccoli for soup toppers, if desired, and then transfer remaining broccoli and veggie and stock mixture to a blender and add the turmeric, almond milk and a pinch of salt and pepper. Blend this mixture on high until it is smooth. Divide the soup among bowls and then add the shredded chicken and broccoli florets.

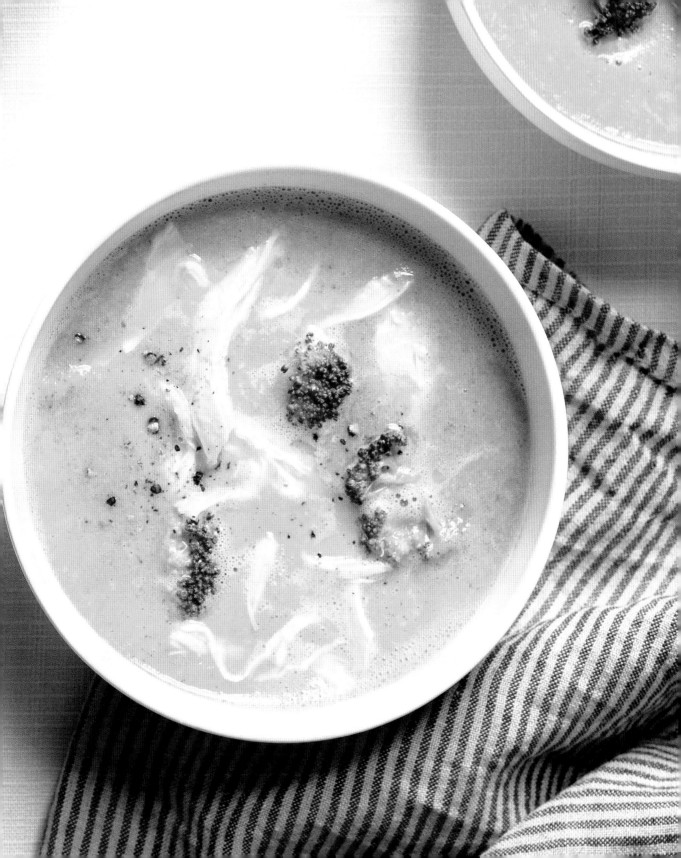

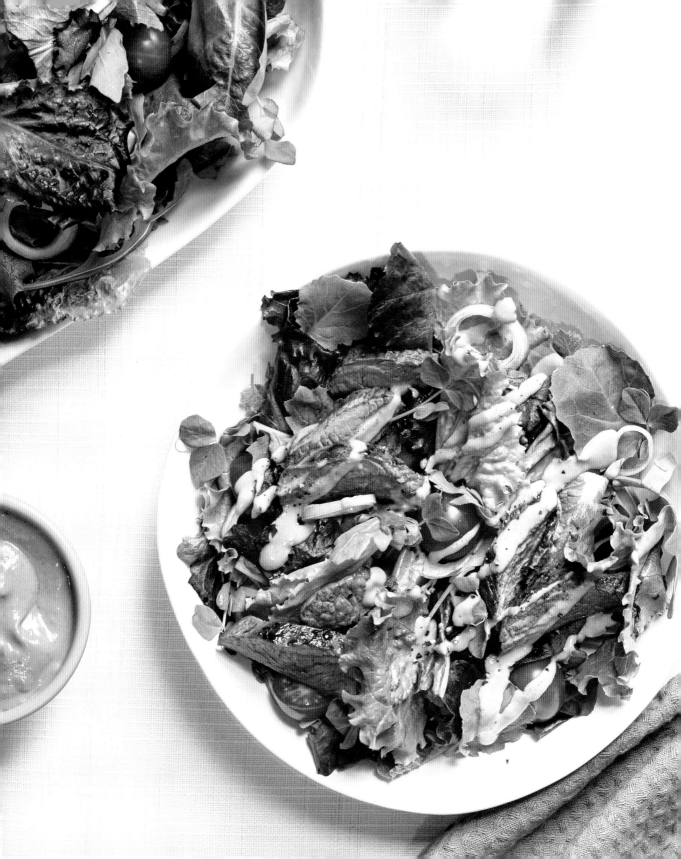

SAVORY STEAK SALAD

Yield: 2 servings

We're all for tasty meals that use simple, healthy ingredients and don't take hours to prepare. All you need here are a few simple items, and you'll have a wonderfully tasty protein- and nutrient-packed meal that really takes very little effort to prepare. Add the green goddess dressing, and you'll add healthy fats, digestive-boosting apple cider vinegar and fresh herbs to the overall nutrition profile of this dish.

1 (8-oz [226-g]) steak (sirloin or filet work well here)

Pinch of salt and pepper

1 tbsp (15 ml) olive oil

3 cups (105 g) mixed salad greens

¼ shallot, sliced thin

½ cup (75 g) cherry tomatoes

GREEN GODDESS DRESSING

1 ripe avocado

3 tbsp (45 g) tahini paste

1 tbsp (15 ml) apple cider vinegar

Juice of 1 lemon

2 tbsp (20 g) shallot, minced

¾ teaspoon salt

3 cups (180 g) packed mixed herbs such as basil, cilantro, tarragon, mint and parsley

¾ cup (180 ml) water

Heat a cast iron skillet over medium heat. Pat the steak dry with a paper towel and season it with a pinch of salt and pepper on each side. Add the olive oil to the hot skillet and then sear the steak for 4 to 5 minutes on each side, until it is well browned and cooked to your liking. A medium steak will be 140°F (60°C), and well done will be 160°F (71°C). Remove the steak from the skillet and allow it to rest for 10 minutes before slicing against the grain.

Meanwhile, make the dressing by adding the avocado, tahini paste, apple cider vinegar, lemon juice, minced shallot, salt, mixed herbs and water to a blender and mix everything on high speed until the dressing is smooth. For a thinner dressing, add more water a few tablespoons at a time until the desired consistency has been reached.

Divide the salad greens between two plates and add the sliced shallots and cherry tomatoes, followed by the steak. Drizzle the salad with green goddess dressing and serve.

Note: dressing can be stored in the refrigerator for 3 days. Some discoloration may occur due to the avocados oxidizing.

CAULIFLOWER RICE TACO BOWL

Yield: 4 servings

A great way to substitute carbs in a meal is to use cauliflower rice. Not only do you give your blood sugar and insulin levels a break by adding cauliflower rice to your meal, but the vegetable also contains the all-essential liver-supporting compound: sulfur. Now spice up your cauliflower rice with these taco bowls!

1 avocado

1½ limes, divided, plus more for serving

⅓–½ cup (80–120 ml) water, divided

1 lb (454 g) lean ground beef

1 tsp cumin

¼ tsp chili powder

3 cups (339 g) cauliflower rice

2 tbsp (2 g) cilantro, chopped, plus more for serving

1 cup (43 g) lettuce

½ cup (35 g) purple cabbage, thinly sliced

½ cup (136 g) pico de gallo

Place the avocado and juice from 1 lime into a food processor or blender and process on high until it is smooth. Add ¼ to ⅓ cup (60 to 80 ml) of water a couple of tablespoons at a time to slightly thin the crema. Place the crema in the refrigerator until it is needed.

Heat a medium-sized skillet over medium-high heat. Cook the ground beef, breaking it into small pieces with a spatula, until it is well browned. Add the cumin, chili powder, and ¼ cup (60 ml) of water and cook for an additional 2 to 3 minutes, and then remove from the heat.

Steam the cauliflower rice for 2 to 3 minutes on the stove, and then stir in the chopped cilantro and the juice of half a lime. Divide the cauliflower rice among four bowls then top it with the ground beef, lettuce, purple cabbage, pico de gallo and avocado crema. Serve with lime wedges and cilantro.

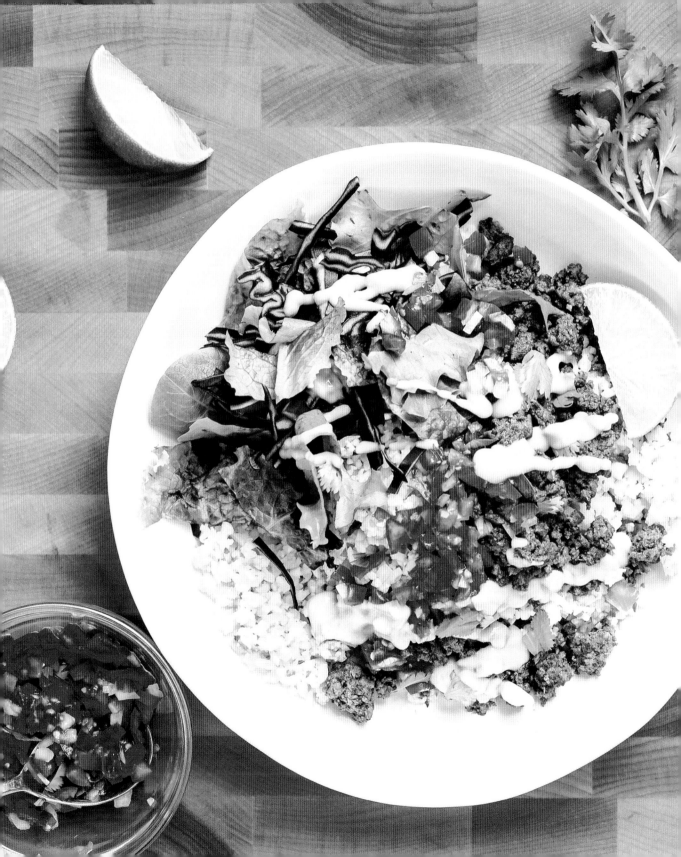

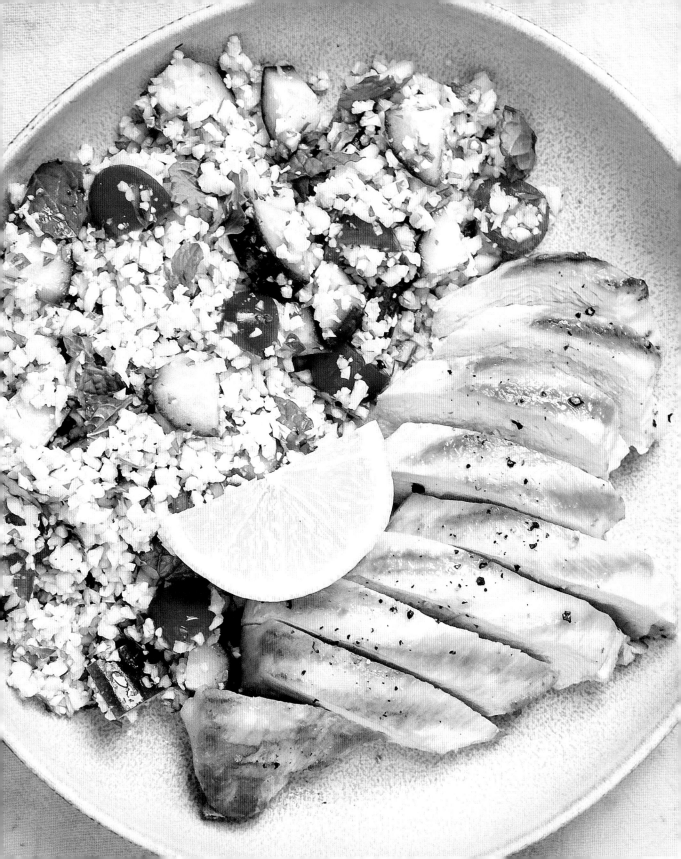

TABBOULEH WITH CHICKEN BREAST

Yield: 2 servings

Need something light and healthy but satisfying and tasty? Let's rustle up a tabbouleh salad with chicken. Tabbouleh is traditionally made with bulgur wheat, but it can be a bit heavy, not only on your stomach, but on the carbs as well. So we have a solution: cauliflower rice. Cauliflower rice is such a great alternative to any starch in a meal. It adds another source of vegetables but gives you the illusion of the carb portion of the meal, so you'll likely not even miss the bulgur. Add a lean source of protein with this combo and you have a quick, easy and light meal that's packed full of flavor.

3 cups (339 g) cauliflower rice

2 Persian cucumbers, diced

1 cup (180 g) cherry tomatoes, diced

¼ cup (16 g) parsley, finely chopped

¼ cup (23 g) roughly chopped mint leaves

3 tbsp (45 ml) olive oil, divided

Juice of 1 lemon

Salt and pepper to taste

2 chicken breasts

Lightly steam the cauliflower rice on the stovetop for 1 to 2 minutes and then transfer it to a bowl to cool. Add the diced cucumber, cherry tomatoes, fresh herbs, 2 tablespoons (30 ml) of olive oil, lemon juice, and salt and pepper to taste. Set the cauliflower rice aside.

Heat a skillet over medium heat and add 1 tablespoon (15 ml) of olive oil. Pat the chicken breasts dry and sprinkle with a pinch of salt and pepper. Cook the chicken for approximately 10 to 12 minutes, flipping it halfway through, until the internal temperature reaches 165°F (74°C). Alternatively, you can cook the chicken breast in the oven for 20 to 22 minutes at 400°F (204°C). Allow the chicken to rest for a couple of minutes before slicing and serving on top of the tabbouleh.

CHICKEN CAESAR KALE SALAD

Yield: 2 servings

Caesar salads are a popular choice for those looking for a healthy but tasty meal. The trouble is, your traditional Caesar salad is packed full of fat and calories under the illusion of many green layers of lettuce. There're simply too many industrial seed oils and gluten-filled croutons for it to be a healthy meal. Now, we don't want you to give up on a good Caesar! We do, however, encourage you to make a few tweaks to suit this new way of eating. Your bases remain crunchy and green, while your dressing becomes a salty sour combo that includes anchovies, garlic, lemon, mayo and mustard. Add a lean source of protein with the chicken and that's that. What more could you want?

SALAD

1 tbsp (15 ml) olive oil

2 chicken breasts

Pinch of salt and pepper

1 head romaine, chopped

1 cup (67 g) baby kale

¼ red onion, sliced thinly

½ cup (75 g) cherry tomatoes, halved

½ greenhouse cucumber, sliced

DRESSING

2 anchovies, minced

1 clove garlic, minced

¼ tsp salt

⅓ cup (80 ml) Paleo-style mayonnaise (see page 93)

2 tsp (10 ml) lemon juice

1 tsp Dijon mustard

½ tsp pepper

Preheat the oven to 400°F (204°C). Heat a cast iron skillet or grill pan over medium heat. Then, add the olive oil. Season the chicken breasts with salt and pepper and then sear them until they are golden brown, for 1 to 2 minutes on medium heat. Flip them over and then transfer the skillet to the oven to finish cooking. The cook time will depend on the thickness of the chicken breast—for thin breasts, begin checking at 10 minutes. Thicker breasts may take up to 15 minutes. Remove the chicken from the oven when the internal temperature reaches 165°F (74°C).

While the chicken is cooking, prepare the dressing. Place the minced anchovies and garlic on a cutting board along with the salt. Using the blade and flat edge of a knife, cut and smash the garlic and anchovies into a paste. Add the paste to a small bowl along with the mayo, lemon juice, Dijon and pepper. Whisk everything together to combine. If the dressing is very thick, add 1 to 2 tablespoons (15 to 30 ml) of water to thin it out.

Divide the romaine and kale between two bowls and top with the onion, tomatoes and cucumber. Slice the chicken and add that to the salads, and then drizzle with the Caesar dressing.

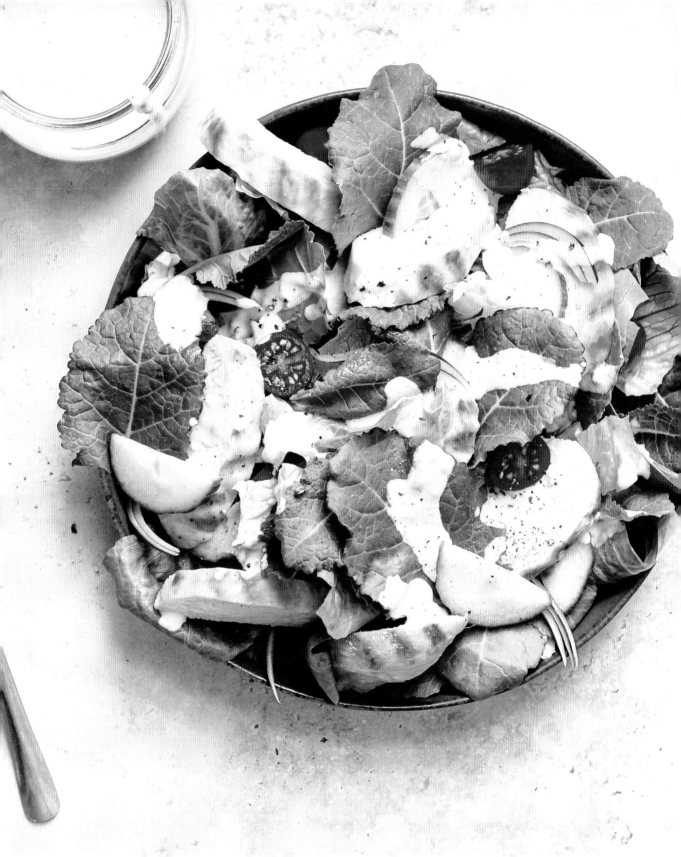

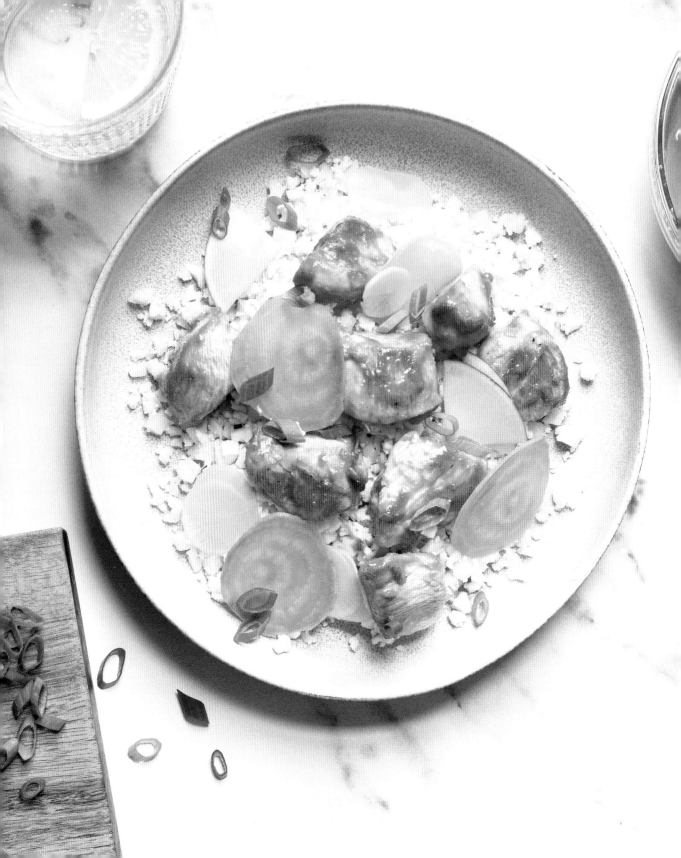

GLAZED CHICKEN & CAULIFLOWER RICE BOWL WITH QUICK PICKLED VEGETABLES

Yield: 2 servings

Gut health is one of our top priorities—optimizing your gut health is one of the key steps in maintaining good health and keeping all of your body systems running as they should. Fermented foods are a great way to include a rich food source for your gut bacteria. It's the gut bacteria that helps to add various nutrients back into your body when they ferment food in your colon. It's why we've included a quick pickled vegetables recipe in this pack. Add them to a lean protein dish like this glazed chicken and low carb cauliflower rice option for an all-around super nutritious, simply delicious, healthy meal.

PICKLED VEGETABLES

1 cup (116 g) thinly sliced root vegetables such as turnips, radishes or beets

⅓ cup (80 ml) apple cider vinegar

½ cup (120 ml) water

1 tbsp (15 ml) honey

½ teaspoon salt

RICE BOWL

1 tbsp (15 ml) olive oil

2 chicken breasts, cut into 2-inch (5-cm) pieces

Pinch of salt and pepper

2 tbsp (30 ml) Dijon mustard

1½ tbsp (22 ml) maple syrup (organic is best)

2 cloves garlic, minced

2 tbsp (30 ml) water

2 cups (226 g) cauliflower rice

2 scallions, thinly sliced

Prepare the pickled vegetables first. Place the thinly sliced vegetables into a shallow bowl. In a small saucepan, heat the apple cider vinegar, water, honey and salt until the honey and salt have dissolved. Pour over the vegetables and set aside while you prepare the rest of the dish.

Heat a cast iron skillet over medium heat and add the olive oil. Season the chicken with a pinch of salt and pepper. Then, add the chicken to the skillet and cook for 10 minutes, stirring halfway through until the chicken is evenly browned on all sides.

While the chicken is cooking, add the mustard, maple syrup, minced garlic and water to a small bowl and whisk to combine. When the chicken is browned on all sides, pour the maple-mustard mixture into the skillet and continue cooking, stirring often until the liquid has thickened and coated the chicken. Remove the chicken from the heat.

In a separate nonstick skillet, heat the cauliflower rice and sauté it for 2 to 3 minutes until it is tender. Divide the rice between the two bowls and then add the chicken and some of the pickled vegetables. Garnish with scallions.

ROASTED SALMON SALAD

Yield: 2 servings

Need a quick, delicious and healthy meal in under 15 minutes? We've got you! It's a salad, but *this* salad has everything you need; it offers healthy fats from the omega 3–rich salmon, an array of vitamins and minerals from the heap of salad greens, various oils and nutrients from the olives and a secret crunch that may surprise you. Don't forget the sweet and sour vinaigrette that takes just seconds to whip up! Gone are those boring salad days. Here's a salad you can look forward to, and a dish that can help you to stay on track with your healthy eating habits, even when you're in a time crunch!

SALAD

2 (4–6 oz [113–170 g]) salmon filets

1 tbsp (15 ml) olive oil

Pinch of salt and pepper

4 cups (140 g) mixed salad greens

¼ cup (30 g) pitted olives

2 tbsp (9 g) pumpkin seeds

SHALLOT VINAIGRETTE

1 tbsp (10 g) minced shallot

1 tsp Dijon mustard

1 tbsp (15 ml) lemon juice

½ tsp honey (local honey is best)

Pinch of salt and pepper

¼ cup (60 ml) olive oil

Preheat the oven to 400°F (204°C). Place the salmon on a parchment-lined baking tray and drizzle with the olive oil and a pinch of salt and pepper. Cook for 8 to 12 minutes or until the internal temperature has reached 145°F (63°C).

Meanwhile, prepare the vinaigrette by whisking together the shallot, mustard, lemon juice, honey, salt and pepper. Slowly whisk in the olive oil.

Divide the salad greens, olives and pumpkin seeds between two bowls. Top with the cooked salmon and drizzle with the shallot vinaigrette.

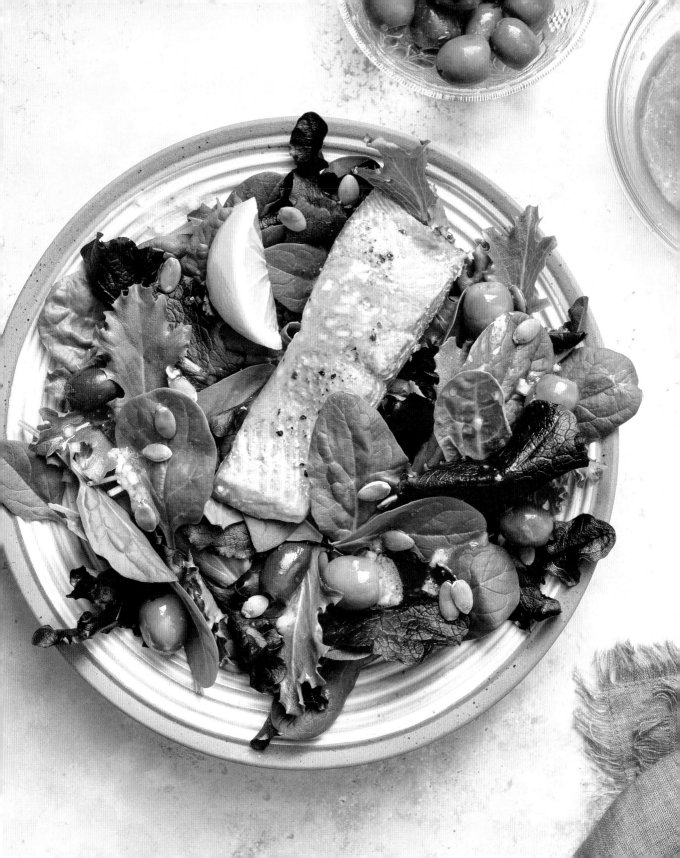

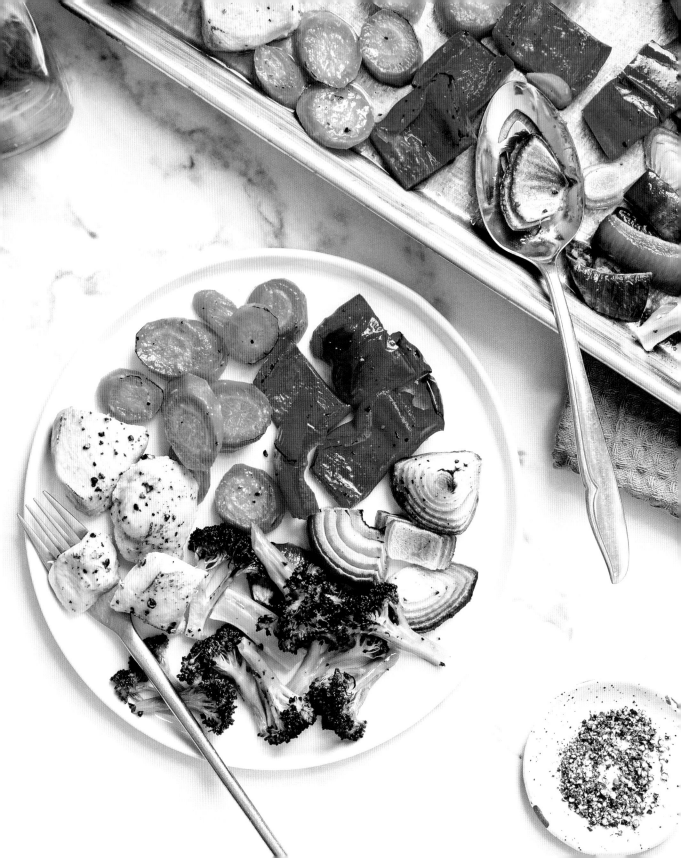

RAINBOW VEGETABLE & CHICKEN TRAY BAKE

Yield: 2–3 servings

Ever heard that you should "eat the rainbow?" Now you'll know how to! With this vegetable and chicken bake, you'll get the colors of the rainbow all in one plate and the nutrients they boast to boot! Packed with flavor and a quick and easy, healthy meal option, this dish will look just as inviting as it tastes.

1 red bell pepper

1 red onion

3 large carrots

1 small head broccoli

3 tbsp (45 ml) olive oil, divided

Salt and pepper

2 chicken breasts

Preheat oven to 400°F (204°C).

Cut the pepper, onion, carrots and broccoli into equally sized pieces approximately 2 inches (5 cm) big. Toss with 2 tablespoons (30 ml) of olive oil and a pinch of salt and pepper and arrange them on a rimmed baking tray.

Cut the chicken breasts into 2-inch (5-cm) pieces and place them on the tray. Drizzle the chicken with the remaining tablespoon (15 ml) of olive oil and a pinch of salt and pepper.

Place the tray of vegetables and chicken in the oven and cook for 15 minutes. Then, turn the oven to broil and cook for an additional 5 to 7 minutes until the vegetables begin to char around the edges and chicken has reached an internal temperature of 165°F (74°C).

ROASTED CARROT & FENNEL SOUP WITH CHICKEN

Yield: 2 servings

Did you know that fennel contains estrogen-balancing compounds? It's true, which is why we include it in this delicious, heart-warming soup recipe. With the added benefits of vitamin A-packed carrots and lean protein from chicken, it's a dish with a great flavor profile that we're sure will be a recurring addition to your weekly menu.

1 lb (454 g) carrots, peeled and halved lengthwise

1 onion, peeled and quartered

½ fennel bulb, sliced into 6 wedges

¼ cup (60 ml) olive oil, plus more for drizzling

Salt and pepper

1 chicken breast

3 cups (720 ml) chicken or vegetable stock

Preheat the oven to 400°F (204°C). Place the carrots, onion and fennel on a rimmed baking sheet and toss with the olive oil and a pinch of salt and pepper. Make a space in the center for the chicken breast. Flip the breast over a couple of times on the tray to coat with olive oil and then place the tray in the oven. Roast for 20 to 25 minutes until the chicken breast has reached 165°F (74°C), flipping the vegetables halfway through. If the vegetables finish before the chicken, carefully remove them from the tray and allow the chicken to finish cooking.

Once cooked, place the vegetables into a blender along with the stock. Blend on high speed until the vegetables and stock are pureed. Transfer the soup back to a pot and gently reheat it while shredding the chicken breast. Add the chicken back to the soup and top with a drizzle of olive oil and some fennel fronds.

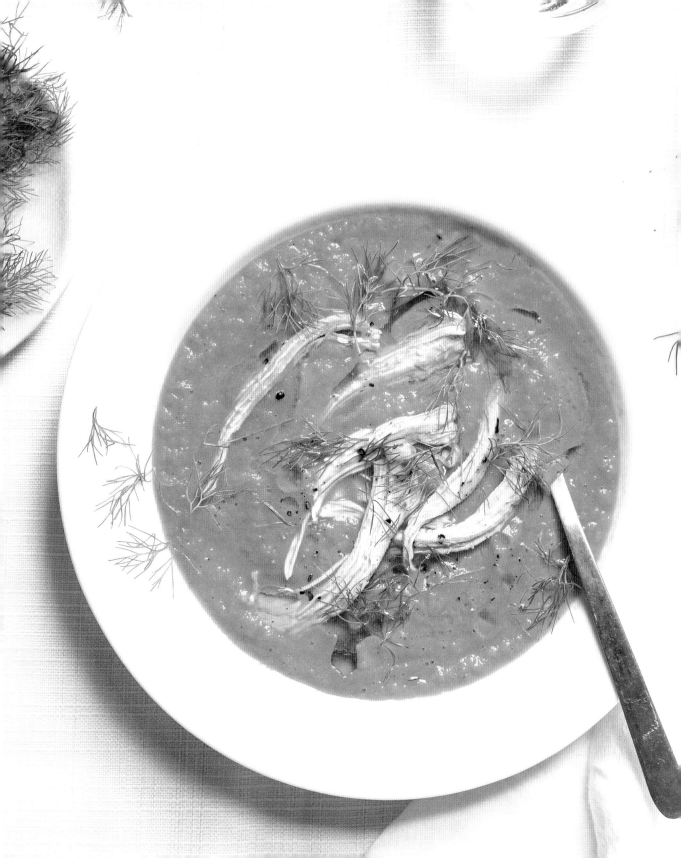

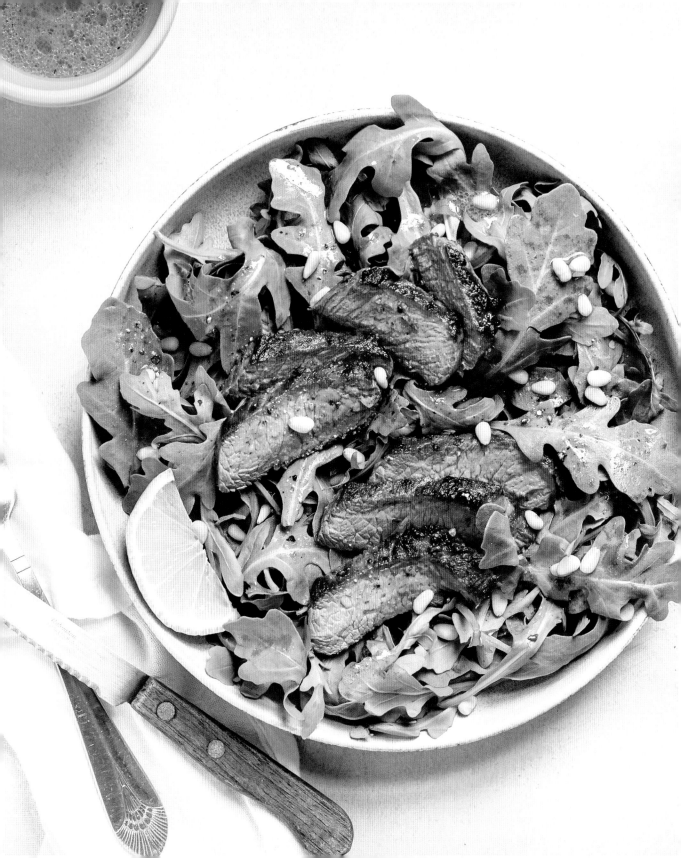

DINNERS

ITALIAN SEARED BEEF SALAD

Yield: 2 servings

Did you know that beef is one of the main readily available sources of iron and vitamin B12 in your diet? Both of these nutrients have important roles in the body, particularly for energy maintenance and feelings of well-being. A simple way to add beef to your diet is to add it to a simple salad. Don't be mistaken, though—there's nothing simple about the flavors here!

Juice of ½ lemon

½ tsp Dijon mustard

2 tbsp (30 ml) plus 1 tsp olive oil, divided

Salt and pepper

1 (1-inch [2.5-cm]) thick sirloin steak, approximately 8 oz (226 g)

3 cups (60 g) arugula

¼ cup (34 g) pine nuts

Prepare the vinaigrette dressing by whisking together the lemon juice, mustard, 2 tablespoons (30 ml) of olive oil and a pinch of salt and pepper. Set this aside.

Heat a cast iron skillet over medium heat. Pat the steak dry and sprinkle with salt and pepper on both sides. Add the remaining teaspoon of olive oil to the pan and then sear the steak for 4 to 5 minutes until it is well browned on each side. The internal temperature for medium rare is 135°F (57°C) and medium is 140°F (60°C). Remove the steak from the heat and allow it to rest for 10 minutes before slicing.

Meanwhile, divide the arugula between the bowls and toss the greens with the vinaigrette and pine nuts. Slice the steak and divide between the bowls.

CHICKEN TORTILLA SOUP

Yield: 4 servings

Soup is a great way to add a whole load of nutrients into one easy-to-digest meal, but many people avoid it because they don't find it filling enough. Here's a way to include soup as a hearty and wholesome meal that's easy on the digestive system in a way that will leave you feeling completely satisfied from a flavor and nutritional perspective.

2 tbsp (30 ml) olive oil, divided

2 poblano peppers, diced

1 onion, diced

½ jalapeño, deseeded and finely diced (optional)

1 (28-oz [792-ml]) jar of fire-roasted tomatoes

6 cups (1.4 L) chicken broth

2 chicken breasts

1 tsp chili powder

1 tsp cumin

Salt and pepper to taste

¼ cup (4 g) chopped cilantro, plus more to garnish

4 medium-sized Paleo tortillas

Lime wedges

Jalapeño slices to serve (optional)

Heat a soup pot over medium heat and add 1 tablespoon (15 ml) of olive oil. Add the poblano peppers, onion and jalapeño to the pot and sauté for 2 to 3 minutes, until the peppers and onion are just tender. Then, add the tomatoes, chicken broth, chicken breasts, chili powder, cumin and a pinch of salt and pepper, and then bring to a simmer. Simmer for 15 to 20 minutes until the chicken breasts are very tender and cooked all the way through. Then, remove the breasts from the pot and transfer them to a cutting board. Use two forks to shred the chicken and then add them back to the pot, along with the chopped cilantro.

Meanwhile, turn the broiler on. Slice the tortillas in half and then cut them into ¼-inch (6-mm) strips. Place them on a baking tray and toss with 1 tablespoon (15 ml) of olive oil and a pinch of salt. Broil for 3 to 5 minutes until they are crisped and browning around the edges.

Divide the soup into bowls and top with a handful of crispy tortillas, cilantro, lime and jalapeño slices, if using.

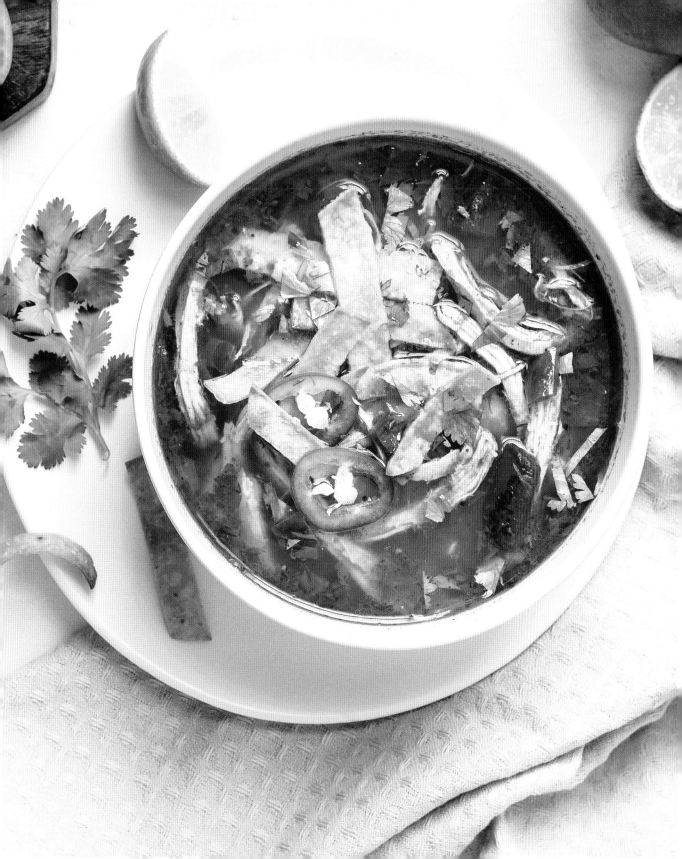

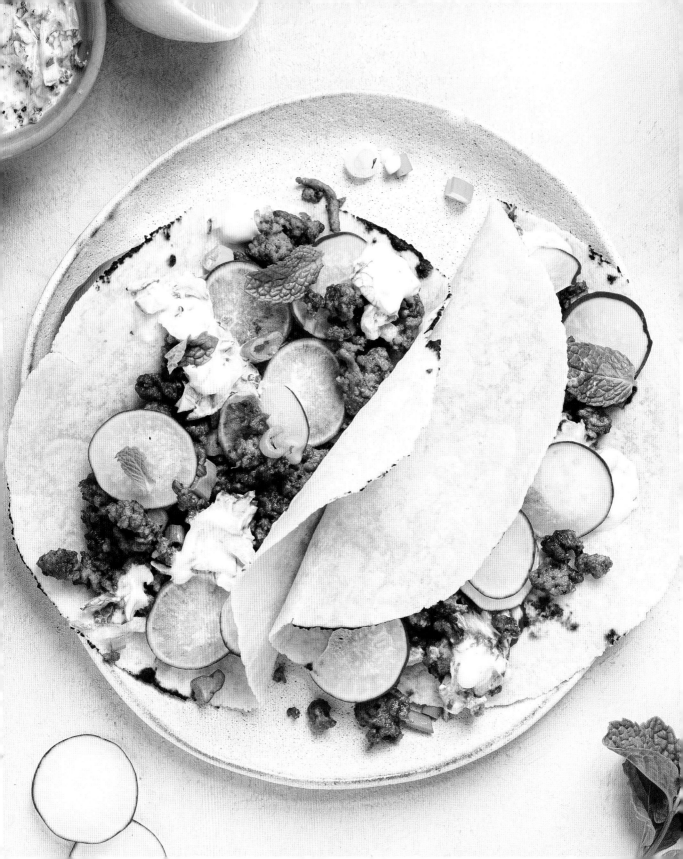

LAMB TACOS WITH PALEO TZATZIKI

Yield: 4 servings

Eating sufficient protein is essential for hormonal balance, and what better way to incorporate protein into your diet than with these succulent, juicy and tangy lamb tacos? It's an easy way to satisfy cravings for fast food favorites, an easy way to prepare a meal and an easy way to keep you on track with eating healthy without feeling like you're missing out.

TZATZIKI

2 Persian cucumbers

Pinch of salt

2 tbsp (30 ml) Paleo-style mayonnaise (see page 93)

¼ tbsp (4 ml) coconut milk

1 tbsp (15 ml) lemon juice

Pinch of salt and pepper

2 tbsp (12 g) chopped fresh mint

TACOS

1 lb (454 g) ground lamb

1 tsp cumin

½ tsp salt

¼ tsp pepper

8 Paleo tortillas

2–3 radishes, thinly sliced

¼ cup (12 g) scallions, sliced

Make the tzatziki by grating the cucumbers and sprinkling them with salt. Let the cucumbers sit for 5 minutes and then squeeze the excess water out. In a small bowl, whisk together the mayonnaise, coconut milk, lemon juice, salt and pepper. Stir in the cucumber and mint and then store in the refrigerator until needed.

Heat a medium-sized skillet over medium heat. Cook the lamb for 7 to 10 minutes, stirring frequently to break it into small pieces. Carefully spoon out the excess fat from the pan and discard it. Add the cumin, salt and pepper while the lamb is cooking. When the lamb is well browned and cooked through, remove it from the heat.

Gently heat the tortillas in a clean skillet and then build the tacos by dividing the lamb, radishes and scallions among the tortillas. Spoon the tzatziki sauce over the tacos.

LEMON PEPPER CHICKEN TRAY BAKE

Yield: 2 servings

Craving some hearty food? We've got you! This lemon pepper chicken bake offers a quick and easy way to prepare a healthy and satisfying home-cooked meal. It's everything you need on one tray: lean protein from the chicken, a complex carbohydrate in the form of potatoes, liver-supporting broccoli and a boost of tangy flavor from the lemons. Enjoy!

2 chicken breasts

Salt and pepper

1 lb (454 g) baby potatoes, halved

2 cups (182 g) broccoli florets

1 lemon, cut into wedges

6 cloves garlic

¼ cup (60 ml) olive oil

Preheat oven to 425°F (218°C). Pat the chicken dry and season it with salt and pepper.

Place the potatoes, broccoli, lemon and garlic on a baking sheet. Pour the olive oil over the vegetables along with a heavy pinch of salt and pepper. Toss the vegetables on the baking tray until they are evenly coated and then clear a spot in the center of the tray for the chicken.

Place the chicken breasts in the center of the baking tray and flip them over a couple of times until they are lightly coated with oil. Transfer them to the oven and bake for 20 to 25 minutes or until the chicken has reached an internal temperature of 165°F (74°C). For a little more color on the chicken, switch to broil for the final 5 minutes of cooking. Remove the baking tray from the oven and squeeze some of the lemon juice over the chicken and vegetables.

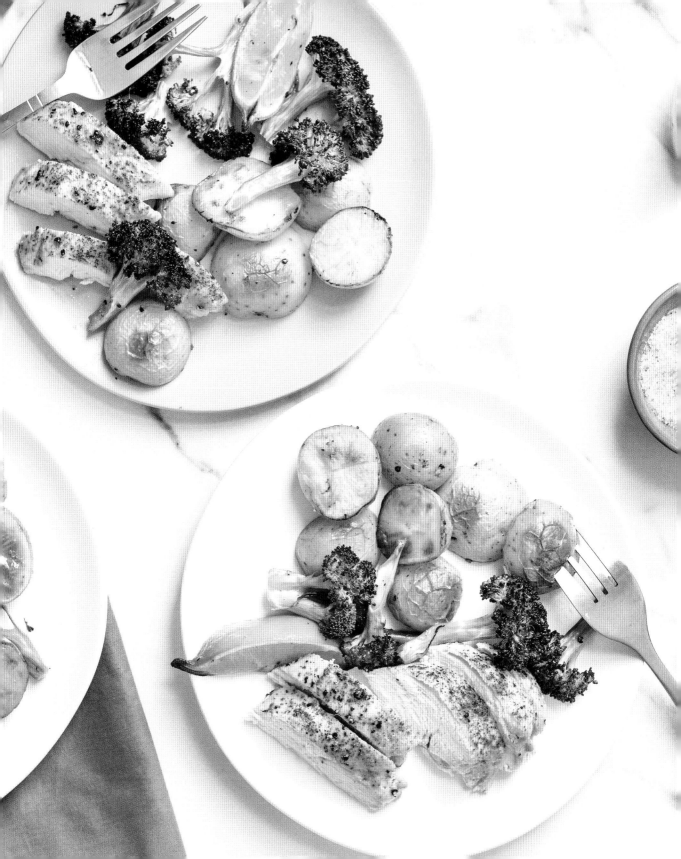

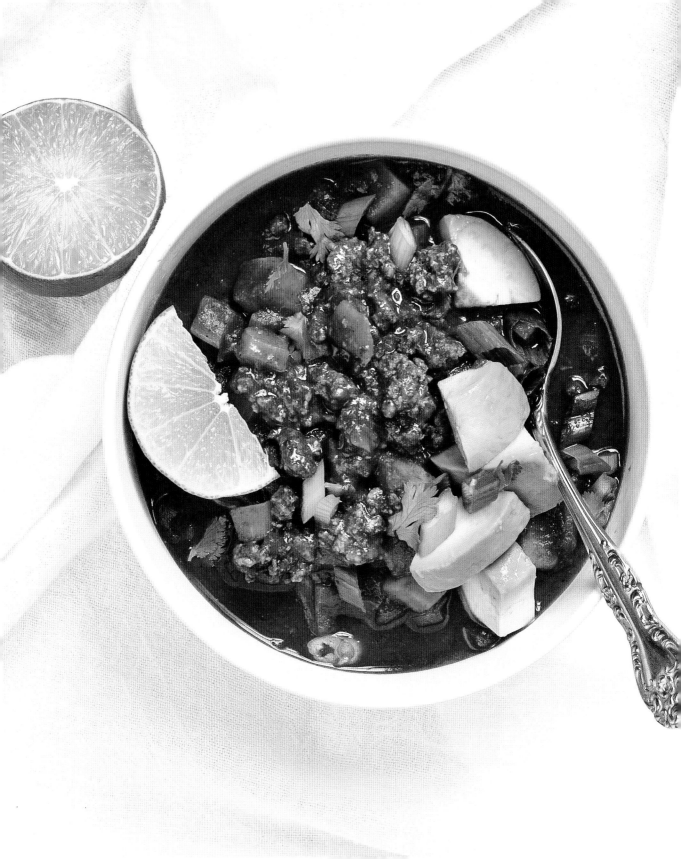

PALEO CHILI

Yield: 4 servings

By now, you'll know that we promote the Paleo diet to support your hormones and your health overall. So why not tap into that style of eating with this scrumptious Paleo chili? Great for warm or cold days, this chili is not only packed with flavor, but it's also a healthy, hearty version of a favorite comfort food.

CHILI

2 tbsp (30 ml) olive oil

1 large sweet potato, diced into ½-inch (1.3-cm) pieces

1 onion, diced

2 celery ribs, diced

2 carrots, diced

1 lb (454 g) of lean ground beef

1 tsp cumin

1 tbsp (8 g) chili powder

1 tsp onion powder

½ tsp oregano

1 tsp salt

1 (14.5-oz [410-ml]) can diced tomatoes

1 (6-oz [168-ml]) can tomato paste

3–4 cups (720–960 ml) vegetable or beef broth

FOR SERVING

1 avocado, diced

¼ cup (4 g) cilantro leaves

¼ cup (12 g) sliced scallions

Lime wedges

Heat a large Dutch oven over medium heat. Add the olive oil and then the diced sweet potato. Cook for 5 to 7 minutes until the potatoes are beginning to color and become a little tender. Add the onion, celery and carrots and cook for an additional 4 to 5 minutes until the onions are slightly translucent and the carrots soften.

Add the ground beef and cook until it is well browned. Add the cumin, chili powder, onion powder, oregano and salt. Stir everything together well and then add the diced tomatoes, tomato paste and broth to the pot. Bring everything to a simmer and then cover the pot and reduce the heat to low. Simmer for at least 30 to 45 minutes or up to 1½ hours to allow all of the flavors to merge. Taste and adjust with salt as necessary. If the chili has become too thick, add water or more broth to thin it.

Serve the chili with diced avocado, cilantro leaves, sliced scallions and lime wedges.

SPAGHETTI SQUASH & MEATBALLS

Yield: 4 servings

The Paleo diet is all about trying to eat whole-some, natural foods, which is why spaghetti squash is such a win. It provides the illusion of a big pasta bowl, without the digestive discomfort or the need to take a nap after eating. It's a great complex carb to add to your diet and, along with the addition of lean beef meatballs, will feel like a real treat.

SPAGHETTI

2 spaghetti squash

2 tbsp (30 ml) olive oil

Pinch of salt

1 (24-oz [672-ml]) jar of sugar-free tomato sauce

½ cup (15 g) spinach

MEATBALLS

1 lb (454 g) lean ground beef

½ onion, minced

2 cloves garlic, minced

¼ cup (16 g) parsley, finely chopped

Preheat the oven to 400°F (204°C). Cut the spaghetti squash in half lengthwise and remove the seeds with a spoon. Place the halves on a rimmed baking tray and drizzle them with the olive oil and a pinch of salt. Cover them with foil and place them in the oven for 40 to 50 minutes or until they are tender and the squash can be separated into spaghetti-like strands easily with a fork.

While the squash is cooking, prepare the meatballs by mixing the lean ground beef, minced onion, minced garlic and chopped parsley in a bowl until everything is thoroughly combined. Pour half the jar of sauce into a 9 x 9–inch (23 x 23–cm) baking dish and then roll the meatballs, aiming for approximately golf ball-sized balls, and place them into the baking dish. Place the spinach into the baking dish, tucking it around the meatballs, and then pour the remaining sauce over the top. Cover them with foil and place the meatballs in the oven with the squash for the last 25 minutes of cooking.

Once the squash has been removed from the oven, turn the broiler on and remove the foil from the meatballs. Cook under the broiler for another 5 to 7 minutes until the sauce is bubbly.

Use a fork to shred the flesh of each squash. You can leave the spaghetti strands in the squash and use that as a serving dish or transfer everything to a bowl. Top the spaghetti squash with meatballs and sauce.

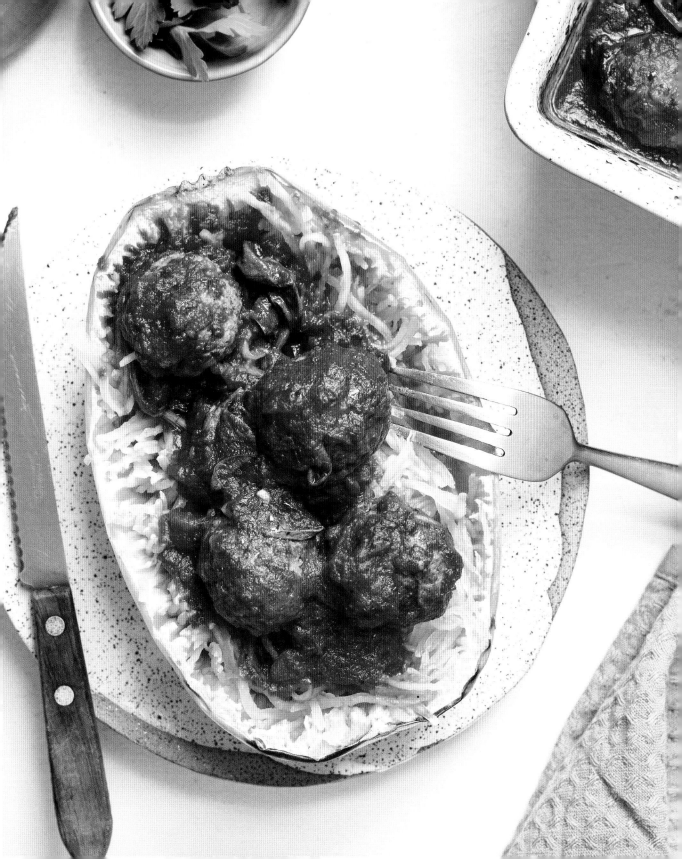

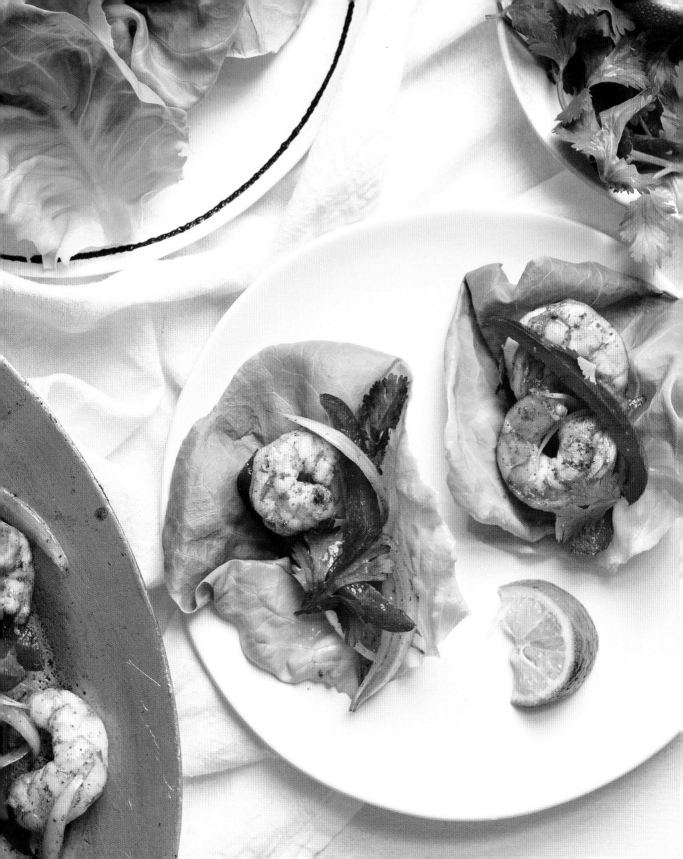

SHRIMP FAJITAS

Yield: 2 servings

Meal inspiration is tough, especially when you're trying a new food plan. That's why we've included these easy-peasy shrimp fajitas. Shrimp cooks quickly, which means dinner will be served in no time. Serve with a hearty helping of leafy greens and you'll have a light yet filling meal in minutes.

1 head butter lettuce or other large leafy green

1 tbsp (15 ml) olive oil

1 bell pepper of any color, sliced thin

½ onion, sliced thin

½ lb (226 g) shrimp, peeled and deveined

½ tsp cumin

½ tsp paprika

½ tsp salt

¼ tsp pepper

1 lime, cut into wedges

Handful of cilantro leaves for serving

Separate the leaves of your lettuce and then wash and dry them well. Place them in the refrigerator until they are needed.

Heat a large skillet over medium heat. Add the olive oil and then the bell pepper and onion and cook for 2 to 3 minutes until the vegetables begin to sweat. Add the shrimp to the pan along with the cumin, paprika, salt and pepper. Cook the shrimp and vegetables, stirring occasionally until the shrimp is bright pink (2 to 3 minutes on each side) and cooked through and the vegetables are tender. The vegetables should take 2 to 3 minutes to cook over medium heat.

Remove the pan from the heat and squeeze two lime wedges over the shrimp and vegetables.

Transfer the shrimp and vegetables to a serving platter and serve alongside the plate of lettuce leaves. Garnish the fajitas with cilantro and more lime if desired.

SAUSAGE, APPLE AND KALE-STUFFED BUTTERNUT SQUASH

Yield: 4 servings

What could be better than a dish filled with fiber, sweetness, complex carbs and protein? Here we add apple and sausage to the rich sweetness of oven-roasted butternut squash for a comfort meal. All of these healthy, nutrient-packed ingredients are there to support the various parts of your body in each of their unique ways.

2 small butternut or honeynut squash, halved and deseeded

2 tbsp (30 ml) olive oil, divided

Salt and pepper

10 sage leaves, 4 whole for garnish and the rest chopped

3 Italian sausage links, casings removed and broken into ½-inch (1.3-cm) pieces

1 tart, firm apple such as Granny Smith or honeycrisp, cored and diced

1 onion, diced

2 cups (134 g) roughly chopped kale

Preheat the oven to 425°F (218°C). Place the cut squash on a baking tray and drizzle it with 1 tablespoon (15 ml) of olive oil, spreading it to make sure the entire surface is lightly coated. Sprinkle the squash with salt and pepper and then flip it so that the cut side is facing down on the baking tray. Roast the squash in the oven for 20 to 25 minutes or until the squash is tender enough to pierce with a fork.

Meanwhile, heat a 10-inch (25-cm) cast iron skillet over medium heat. Heat the remaining 1 tablespoon (15 ml) of olive oil and fry the 4 whole sage leaves until they are crisped, approximately 1 minute. Transfer the sage to a paper towel and add the sausage to the pan. Cook the sausage until it is browned on all sides, for 5 to 7 minutes. Add the diced apple and onion to the pan with a pinch of salt and pepper and cook until the apple and onion just begin to soften, about 3 minutes. Add the kale and chopped sage to the pan and toss until the kale has wilted.

At this point, the squash should be tender. Remove it from the oven and use a spoon to scoop some of the flesh out, leaving a 1-inch (2.5-cm) border. Reserve the squash for another use. Fill the cavity with the sausage filling and return the squash to the oven. Turn the oven to broil and cook the squash for another 4 to 5 minutes to heat everything through. Remove the stuffed squash from the oven and allow it to cool slightly before serving. Garnish with the reserved sage.

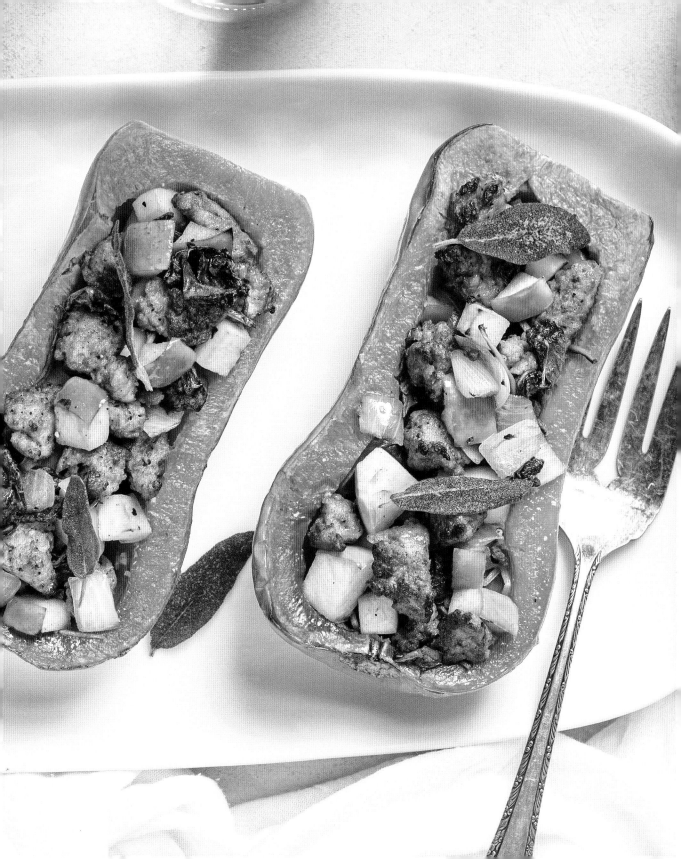

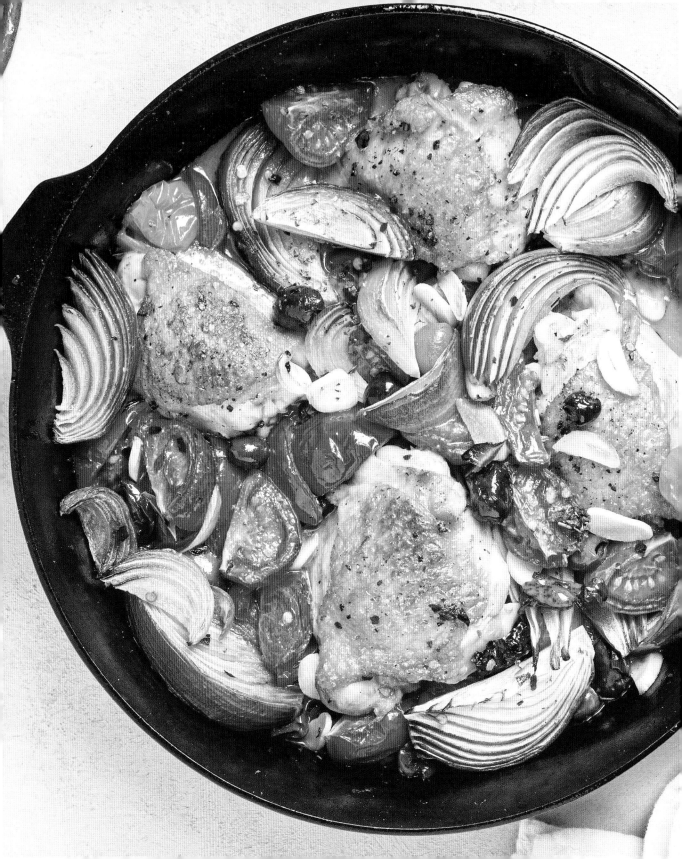

MEDITERRANEAN SKILLET CHICKEN

Yield: 4 servings

One of the most well-studied diets across the entire globe is the Mediterranean diet. It consists of many specific anti-inflammatory foods, full of color and rich in important nutrients. Here, we've focused on the deep reds and purples! In this dish, you're bound to get the anti-inflammatory and antioxidant properties of lycopene from the tomatoes, quercetin from the onions and oleuropein from the olives, all on top of health-boosting garlic, oregano and pepper flakes. Pair that with a lean protein source of chicken breast and serve with a starch-free option such as cauliflower rice as a Paleo protein for a perfectly Mediterranean meal.

4 skin-on, bone-in chicken thighs

Salt and pepper

2 tbsp (30 ml) olive oil

1 large or 2 small red onions, cut into ½-inch (1.3-cm) wedges

1 pint (298 g) cherry tomatoes, halved

⅓ cup (40 g) mixed, pitted olives

4 cloves garlic, sliced

1 tsp oregano

½ tsp red pepper flakes

Preheat the oven to 400°F (204°C). Pat the chicken dry and season it with salt and pepper.

Heat a 10-inch (25-cm) cast iron skillet over medium-high heat. Add the olive oil and place the chicken, skin-side down into the skillet. Sear until a deep golden-brown color is achieved, for approximately 5 minutes. Flip the chicken and add the red onions, cherry tomatoes, pitted olives, garlic, oregano and red pepper flakes to the skillet. Season lightly with salt and pepper and transfer the chicken to the oven.

Bake for 15 to 20 minutes or until the internal temperature of the chicken is 165°F (74°C).

Remove the chicken from the oven and serve. This dish pairs well with grain- and legume-free pasta or cauliflower rice. For grain- and legume-free pasta, we like the company Capello's.

TURKEY MEATBALL SOUP

Yield: 4 servings

If you're tired of eating chicken, give turkey a try. It's also a good alternative to red meat, but has the same versatility, like these tasty turkey meatballs. Using almond flour, we keep these meatballs completely gluten-free, and we add parsley as a little punch of flavor and for its liver-supporting properties. While you can serve them with any meal or even eat them as a quick snack, we love them with this vegetable-rich soup as a base. This easy chicken broth and vegetable soup contains even more nutrients to help your liver to detox, which comes in the form of carrots, spinach and celery.

MEATBALLS

1 lb (454 g) ground turkey

2 tbsp (8 g) chopped parsley

½ cup (64 g) almond flour

1 egg

1 tsp salt

½ tsp pepper

1 clove garlic, minced

1 tbsp (15 ml) olive oil

SOUP

3 tbsp (45 ml) olive oil, divided, plus more for drizzling

1 onion, diced

2 celery ribs, diced

2 carrots, peeled and diced

Pinch of salt

8 cups (1.9 L) chicken broth

2 cups (60 g) spinach or roughly chopped kale

½ cup (26 g) fresh dill, for garnish

To make the turkey meatballs, place the ground turkey, chopped parsley, almond flour, egg, salt, pepper and minced garlic into a medium-sized bowl and use your hands to mix everything together until the mixture is uniform. Form them into golf ball–sized meatballs and set them aside on a tray.

Heat 2 tablespoons (30 ml) of olive oil in a soup pot and gently sauté the onion, celery and carrots with a pinch of salt until just tender, for 2 to 3 minutes. Add the chicken broth and allow everything to come to a simmer.

Meanwhile, heat a large skillet over medium heat and drizzle in 1 tablespoon (15 ml) of olive oil. Sear the meatballs for 1 to 2 minutes until they are well browned on all sides and then transfer them to the simmering soup. Allow them to simmer for at least 15 minutes to ensure the meatballs have cooked through and then add the spinach and cook for another 3 to 5 minutes until it is wilted. Serve the soup with a drizzle of olive oil and a small handful of fresh dill.

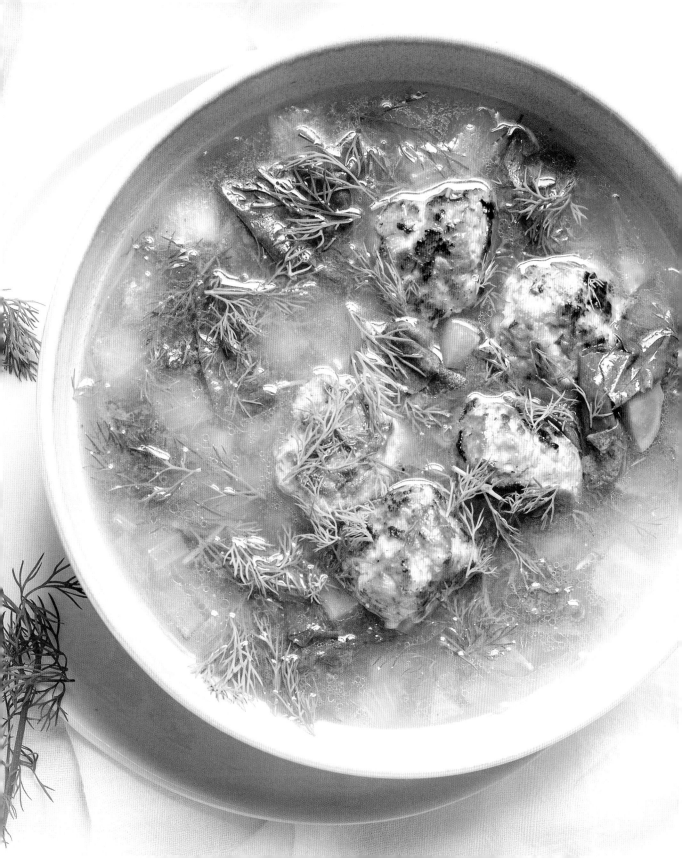

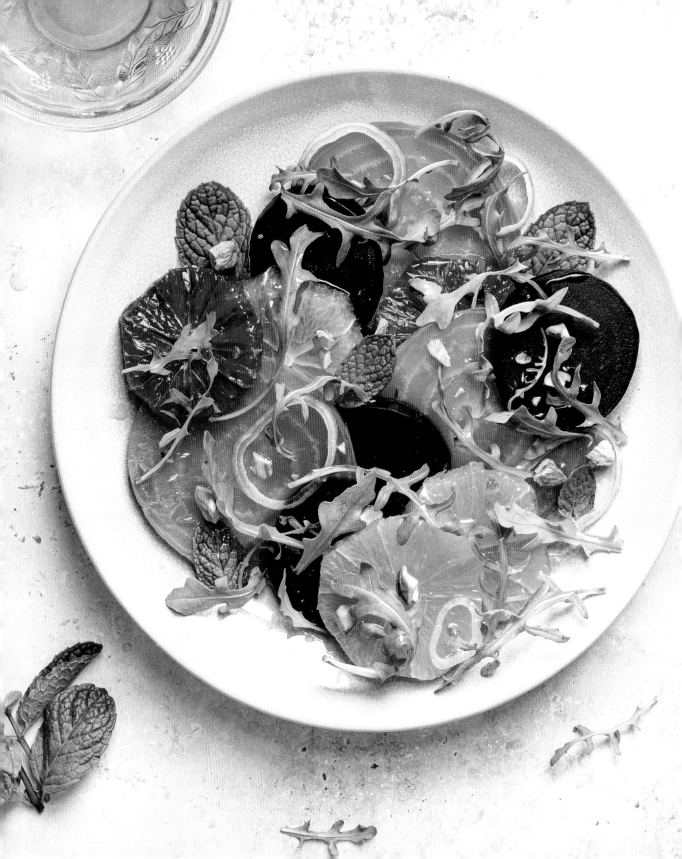

SIDES

BEET & ORANGE SALAD

Yield: 2 servings

It's not only the bright colors of deep red, orange and green that will get you excited about this salad—it's the nutritional value it'll bring to your meal, too! Beets are packed with nutrients. They contribute to brain, digestive and heart health, and they're highly anti-inflammatory. Boost all of this with the richness of vitamin C from the oranges, the bitterness of the greens and invigorating properties of mint and you have the perfect salad. While salad is normally a side, this one will definitely steal the show!

2 beets, any color

2 oranges, navel, blood or other

¼ shallot, sliced into rings

½ cup (10 g) baby arugula

¼ cup (25 g) pistachios or walnuts

Small handful of mint leaves

2 tbsp (30 ml) olive oil

Pinch of salt

Preheat the oven to 400°F (204°) degrees. Scrub the beets (remove greens if there are any) and wrap them tightly in aluminum foil. Place the beets on a baking tray and roast them for 40 minutes to an hour, until a fork can easily pierce the beet. Allow them to cool and then use a paper towel to gently rub away the skins. Slice into ¼-inch (6-mm) rounds and divide them between two plates.

Cut both ends from the oranges and then use a sharp knife to remove all of the skin and pith. Slice into ¼-inch (6-mm) rounds, removing seeds as you work. Divide the oranges between two plates, along with the beets.

Add the shallots, baby arugula, nuts and mint leaves to the plates and then drizzle the salad with the olive oil and add a pinch of salt.

AVOCADO & CITRUS SALAD

Yield: *2 servings*

Here you have a tasty and hormone-friendly combo! Put avocado and oranges together and what do you get? A combination of healthy fats and fiber, as well as a boost of vitamin C to help combat stress. We hope you enjoy this flavorful and tangy salad as much as we do!

2 oranges (blood, navel or Cara Cara work well)

1 tsp honey

2 tbsp (30 ml) olive oil

Pinch of salt and pepper

1 ripe avocado, sliced

¼ cup (40 g) hemp seeds

½ cup (99 g) microgreens or sprouts

Small handful of mint leaves

Remove the peel from both oranges with a knife, leaving no pith behind. Then, slice the oranges into ¼-inch (6-mm) rings. Squeeze the juice from the peels into a small bowl until you have 2 tablespoons (30 ml). Then, whisk in the honey, olive oil and a pinch of salt and pepper to make a vinaigrette.

Arrange the avocado and oranges on plates and then top them with the hemp seeds, microgreens and mint leaves. Drizzle the salad with 2 tablespoons (30 ml) of the vinaigrette (you won't need to use all of it—any remaining dressing can be stored in the refrigerator for a week).

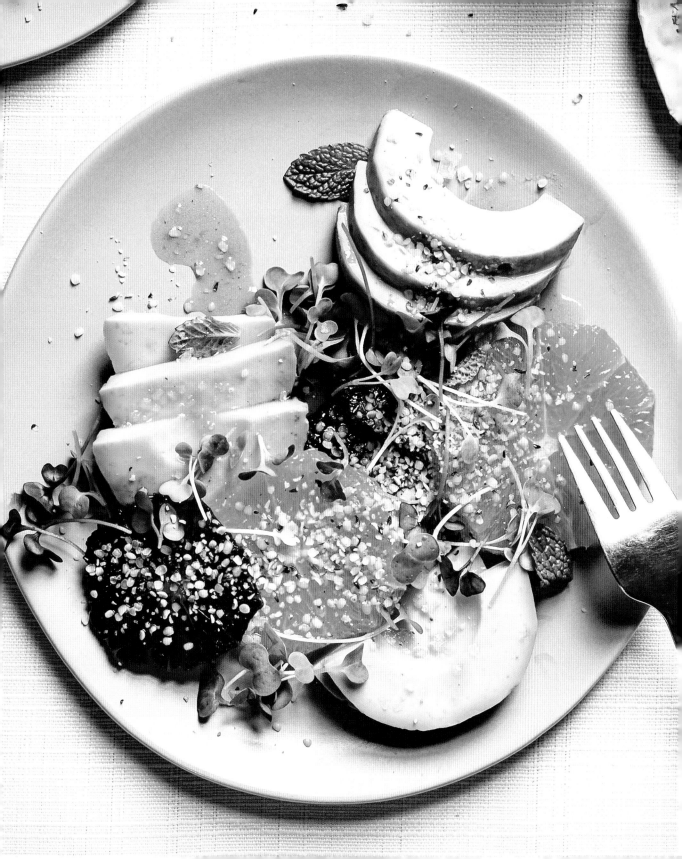

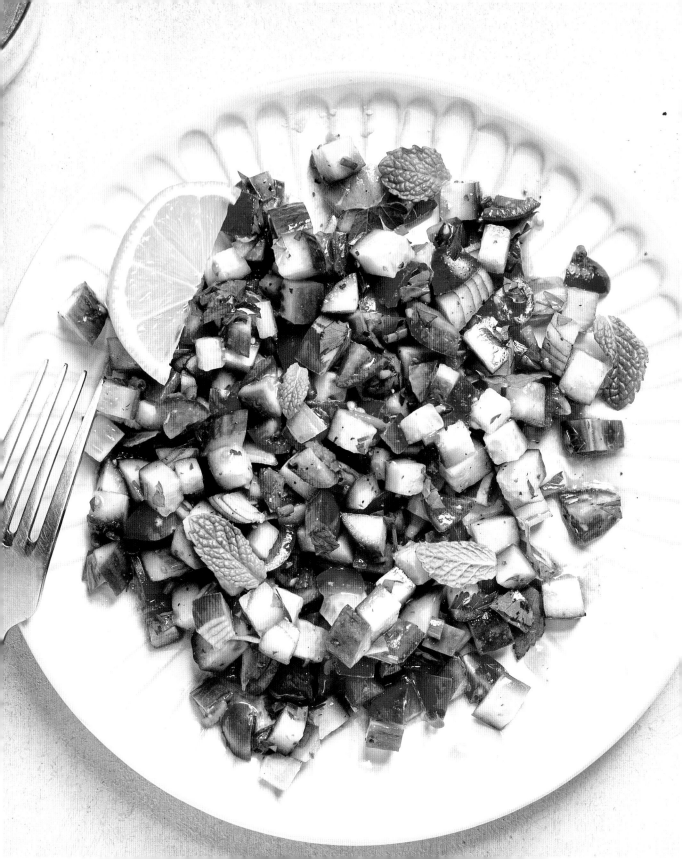

HERBY TOMATO & CUCUMBER SALAD

Yield: 3–4 servings

Fresh herbs are a must in your diet if you're trying to manage your health. The bitterness they bring to your palate is a fantastic way to stimulate your digestive system, and along with that, they all provide their own unique nutritional profiles and benefits. You can try this fresh herb and cucumber salad as a side to any dish!

Dice the cucumber, tomatoes and onion into approximately ¼-inch (6-mm) pieces. Place them into a large bowl and toss them with the basil, parsley, chives, dried oregano, olive oil, lemon juice and a pinch of salt and pepper. This pairs well with the Mediterranean Skillet Chicken (page 129) because the crisp tanginess of this salad keeps with the Mediterranean theme.

3 Persian cucumbers

1 pint (298 g) cherry tomatoes

½ red onion

¼ cup (10 g) basil, roughly chopped

2 tbsp (8 g) parsley, roughly chopped

2 tbsp (6 g) chives, thinly sliced

½ tsp dried oregano

2 tbsp (30 ml) olive oil

Juice of ½ lemon

Pinch of salt and pepper

ROASTED ASPARAGUS WITH CASHEW SAUCE

Yield: 2 servings

Look no further than this saucy asparagus recipe for a tasty and health-boosting side. Asparagus contains compounds that help improve hormone balance, improve body water balance, prevent urinary tract infections and more. Topped with a creamy cashew sauce, you're guaranteed to get some amazing health benefits from this dish.

ASPARAGUS

1 bunch asparagus, ends trimmed

1 tbsp (15 ml) olive oil

Pinch of salt and pepper

CASHEW SAUCE

1 cup (146 g) cashews, soaked overnight

1 clove garlic, minced

Zest and juice of 1 lemon

1 tbsp (5 g) nutritional yeast

2 tsp (10 ml) Dijon mustard

½ tsp salt

¼ tsp pepper

¼ tsp turmeric

⅛ tsp cayenne pepper (optional)

½ cup (120 ml) water

Preheat the oven to 425°F (218°C) with a sheet pan inside. Toss the asparagus with olive oil, salt and pepper and then place them on the sheet tray, evenly spaced. Cook the asparagus for 7 to 10 minutes until they are tender.

Meanwhile, make the cashew sauce by blending together the cashews, minced garlic, lemon zest and juice, nutritional yeast, Dijon mustard, salt, pepper, turmeric, cayenne pepper and water on high until the sauce is creamy. For a thick sauce, use only a ½ cup (120 ml) of water. You can add a ¼ cup (60 ml) water or more to thin the sauce out to a drizzling consistency.

Place ½ cup (120 ml) of the cashew sauce on a platter and arrange asparagus on top. The remaining sauce can be refrigerated and used for up to 5 days.

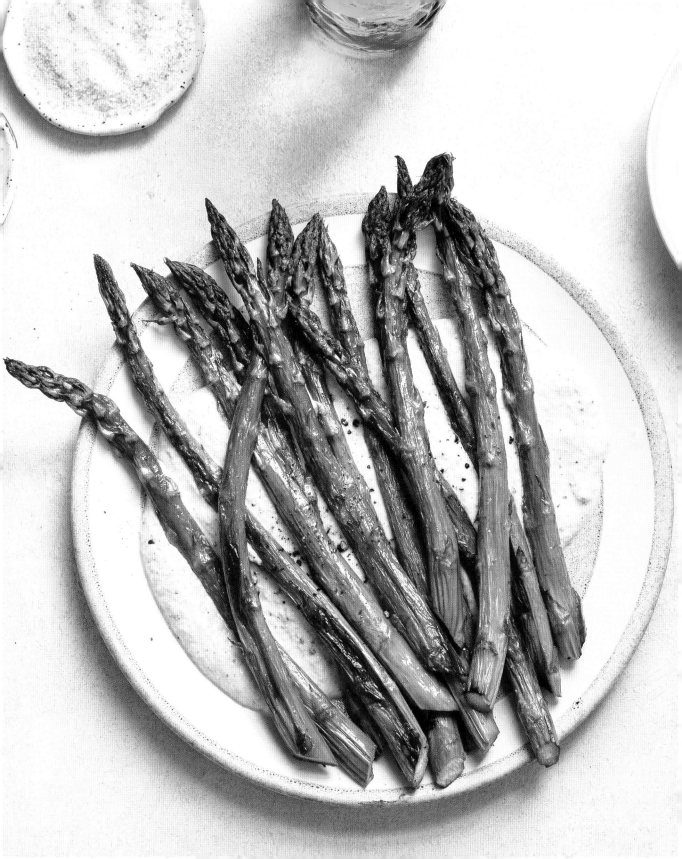

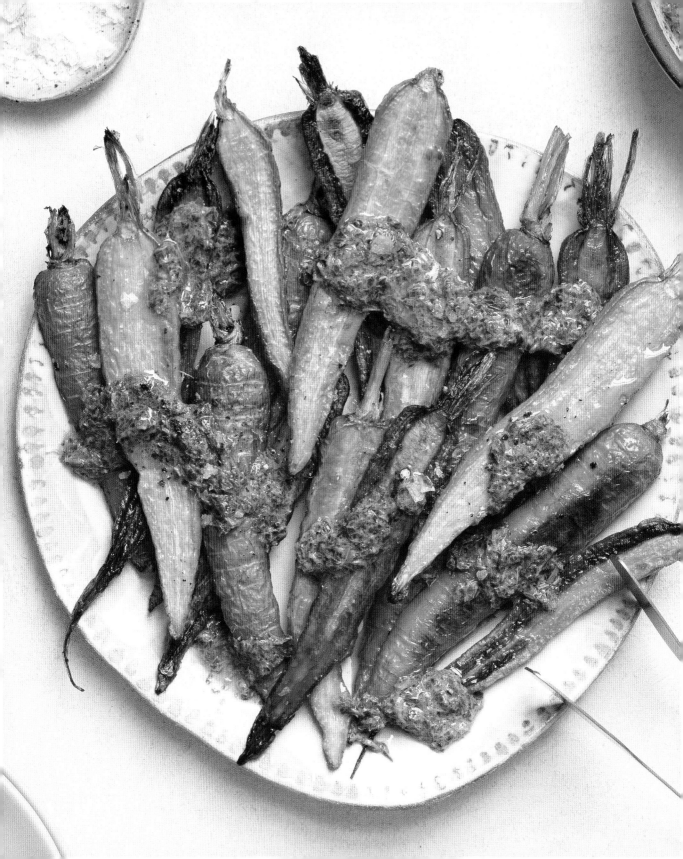

ROASTED CARROTS WITH CREAMY HERB DRESSING

Yield: 2 servings

Raise your hand if you grew up eating mushy, over-boiled carrots that had a grey tinge to them. Now say goodbye to bland carrots for good. Roasting these little roots not only preserves some of their crisp, but also brings out their natural sweetness, which is oh-so-wonderfully complemented by the fresh herb dressing. Carrots? Who knew they could taste so good!

ROASTED CARROTS

1 bunch carrots, washed and tops removed

2 tbsp (30 ml) olive oil

Pinch of salt and pepper

DRESSING

1 egg yolk

½ cup (120 ml) olive oil

1 tbsp (15 ml) apple cider vinegar

1½ cups (90 g) fresh leafy herbs such as chives, parsley, mint and basil

Pinch of salt and pepper

Preheat the oven to 425° (218°C) with a sheet tray inside. If your carrots are very large, cut them in half. Otherwise, leave them whole. Toss the carrots with the olive oil and a pinch of salt and pepper and place them evenly spaced apart on the hot sheet tray. Roast the carrots for 12 to 15 minutes, tossing them once halfway through. The carrots should be browned and tender, but not mushy.

While the carrots are roasting, make the dressing. Place the egg yolk into a small food processor and slowly drizzle in the olive oil while the processor is running. It should become thick and emulsified. Open the processor and add the apple cider vinegar, fresh herbs and a pinch of salt and pepper, and then mix them on high until they are well blended and no large pieces of herbs remain.

When the carrots have finished cooking, transfer them to a platter and dollop the herb dressing over them. Extra dressing can be saved in the refrigerator for up to 3 days.

DESSERTS

BAKED PUMPKIN PUDDING

Yield: 6–8 servings

When you're watching your hormones, you wouldn't dare eat pudding now, would you? Well, why not? We're not talking about the sugar- and fat-laden varieties. We're talking about this delightful pumpkin pudding that is sure to ease those cravings while adding loads of nutritional benefits such as vitamin A, K, C and the minerals copper, magnesium and iron to your diet.

1 (15-oz [425-ml]) can pumpkin puree

1 (15-oz [425-ml]) can coconut milk

¼ tsp salt

2 tsp (4 g) pumpkin pie spice

1 tsp ground ginger

½ cup (120 ml) maple syrup

2 eggs

2 egg yolks

Preheat the oven to 325°F (163°C). Add the pumpkin puree, coconut milk, salt, pumpkin spice, ground ginger, maple syrup, whole eggs and egg yolks to a blender and blend everything together on high until they are smooth and thoroughly blended. Pour the contents of blender into an 8 x 8–inch (20 x 20–cm) baking dish.

Place the baking dish in the oven and bake for 35 to 40 minutes until the edges have puffed and the center is no longer jiggly.

Serve your baked pumpkin pudding warm or chilled.

Note: The pudding can be baked in individually sized ramekins. Begin checking for doneness at 15 minutes.

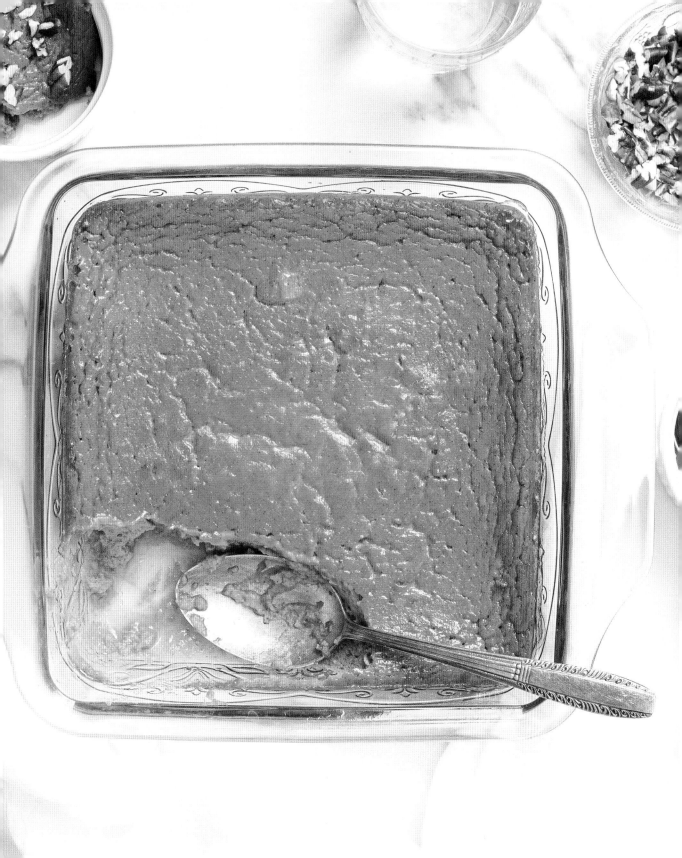

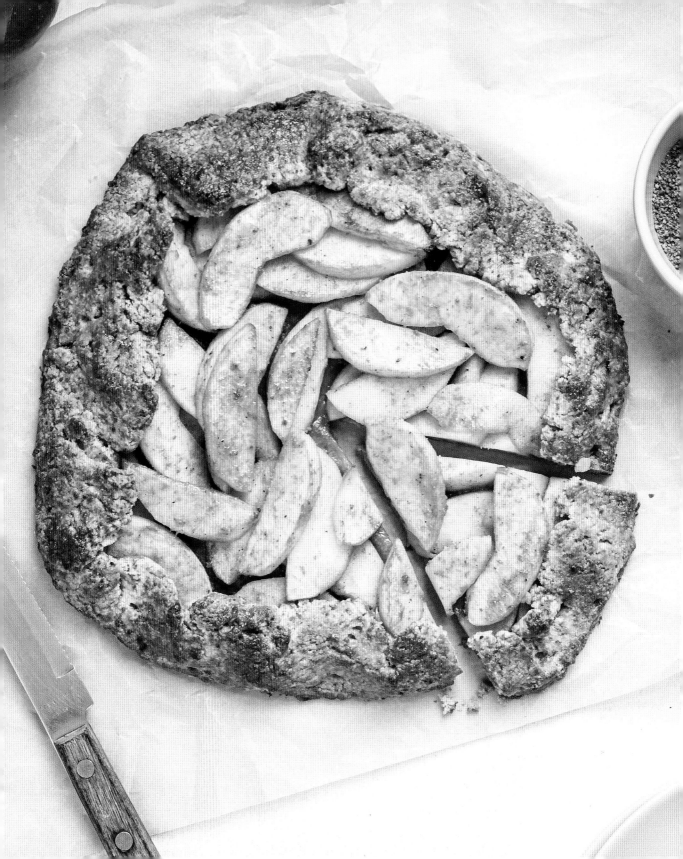

APPLE GALETTE

Yield: 6–8 servings

This deliciously nutritious apple galette has the sweetness of a traditionally made galette, but with a fraction of the sugar, none of the refined flours and the addition of a couple of health-boosting spices such as ginger, nutmeg and/or cinnamon. Ginger is great for the digestive system and holds anti-inflammatory benefits, while cinnamon is great for blood sugar control.

CRUST

¼ cup (60 ml) coconut oil, chilled

1½ cups (192 g) almond flour

½ cup (68 g) + 1 tbsp (8 g) tapioca flour, plus more for dusting

¼ tsp salt

¼ cup (48 g) coconut sugar

1 egg, whisked

FILLING

2 tart firm apples such as honey crisp, peeled, cored and sliced into ¼ inch pieces

½ tsp nutmeg or cinnamon

½ tsp ginger

Pinch of salt

Zest of 1 lemon

Juice of ½ lemon

2 tbsp (24 g) coconut sugar, plus more for sprinkling

1 egg to brush

Cut cold coconut oil into small ¼-inch (6-mm) pieces (you can also use silicone miniature ice trays to make the perfect size) and place them into the freezer for 10 minutes. In a medium-sized bowl, whisk together the almond flour, tapioca flour, salt and coconut sugar. Using your fingers or a pastry cutter, work the very cold coconut oil into the dry ingredients until the pieces are no bigger than lentils. Stir the egg into the mixture until it comes together into a dough, and then knead a couple of times to ensure that no dry spots remain. Wrap the dough in plastic and place it in the refrigerator for an hour and up to overnight.

Preheat the oven to 400°F (204°C) and roll the chilled dough out into a large circle on a piece of parchment, sprinkling it with tapioca flour as you go to prevent sticking. If the edges begin to crack, just squeeze them back together with your hands and keep rolling. The circle should reach approximately 15 inches (38 cm) in diameter and be ¼-inch (6-mm) thick. Transfer the parchment with the dough on it to a baking tray and place it in the refrigerator while you make the filling.

In a large bowl, toss together the apples, nutmeg or cinnamon, ginger, salt, lemon zest and juice and coconut sugar, and then place them in the center of the dough, leaving a 1-inch (2.5-cm) border. Carefully fold the edges up over the apples, squeezing together any areas that are cracking. Be gentle, as this dough can be fragile.

Brush the edges of the dough with egg wash and sprinkle with coconut sugar.

Place the galette in the oven and bake for 18 to 20 minutes or until the crust is well browned.

AVOCADO CHIA PUDDING

Yield: 2–3 servings

We're big into healthy puddings and treats! There's no reason you can't enjoy your food when you're trying to incorporate more healthy ingredients. You can absolutely maximize on the nutritious foods you're eating! Here's a smart way to do so: use chia seeds and avocado in one dish. Get the healthy fats from the avocado and an array of vitamins and minerals from the chia seeds. Top it with toasted coconut and berries and you have a deluxe and delicious yet nutritious pudding. Be sure to make this ahead of time, as it needs some time to set, but it will be worth the wait!

Scoop out the contents of the avocado, and add it to a blender, along with the almond or coconut milk, maple syrup, lemon juice and salt. Puree the mixture until it is smooth.

Transfer the avocado mixture to a bowl and stir in the chia seeds. Refrigerate for an hour or more to allow the chia seeds to plump and for the pudding to set. Due to the avocados, this will eventually discolor, so it's best eaten within 24 hours. To make it extra decadent, enjoy the pudding with some berries and coconut flakes on top!

CHIA PUDDING

1 avocado

1 cup (240 ml) almond or coconut milk

3 tbsp (45 ml) maple syrup

Juice of ½ lemon

Pinch of salt

¼ cup (41 g) chia seeds

OPTIONAL TOPPINGS

Berries

Toasted unsweetened coconut flakes

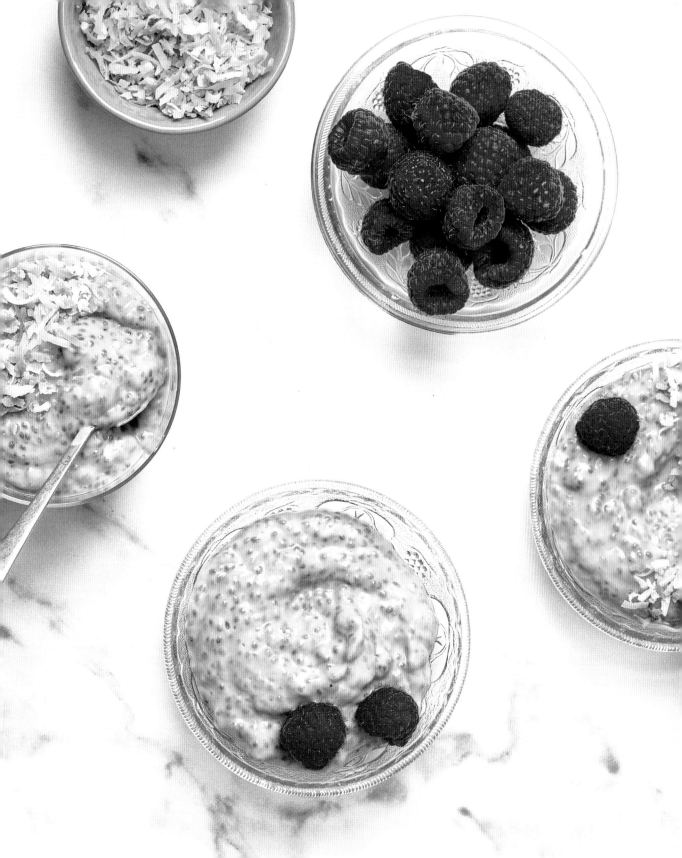

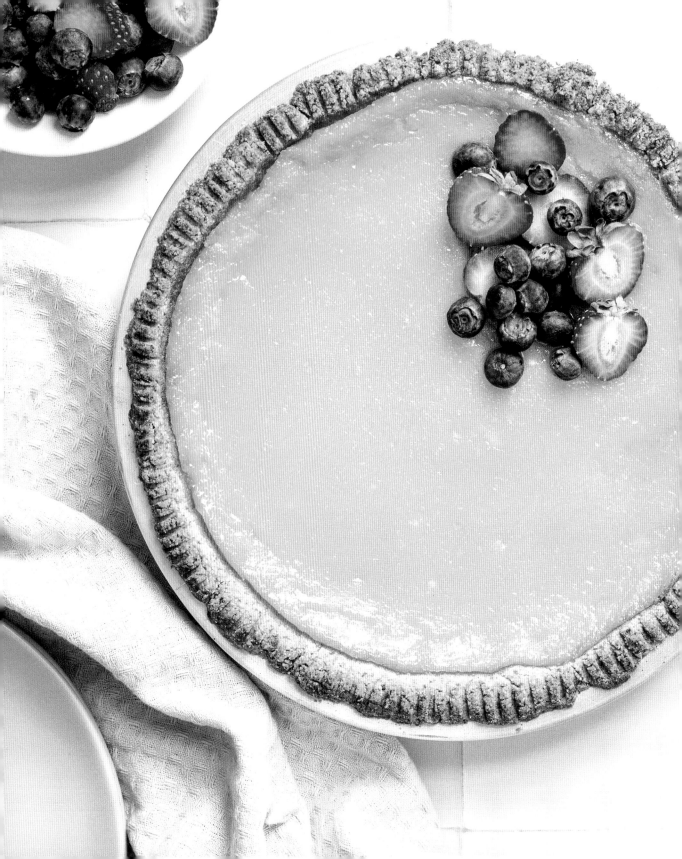

LEMON TART

Yield: 1 (9-inch [23-cm]) tart

Did you know that simply smelling the scent of lemons can boost the release of happy hormones and lower your stress levels? Well, you're sure going to benefit from this aspect when you're making this gloriously sour lemon tart. Lemon juice is also a rich source of vitamin C, which is a vitamin that's super important for balancing out your stress hormones. So, not only will you feel good making and eating this tart, but you can also rest assured that it's good for your body, too.

CRUST

2 cups (256 g) almond flour

¼ cup (32 g) coconut flour

2 tbsp (24 g) coconut sugar

Pinch of salt

¼ cup (60 ml) coconut oil, melted

1 egg, lightly beaten

FILLING

1 cup lemon juice (from 5–7 lemons)

Zest of 3 lemons

¾ cup (180 ml) honey

4 tbsp (56 g) grass-fed butter

¼ cup (60 ml) coconut oil

Prepare the crust by mixing the almond flour, coconut flour, coconut sugar and a pinch of salt together in a medium-sized bowl. Make a well in the center and add the coconut oil and egg. Stir everything together until it forms a dough for the crust, and then transfer it to a 9-inch (23-cm) tart pan or pie tin and carefully press the crust into the pan to form an even layer across the bottom and sides. If you are using a pie tin, you can use a fork to create a crimped rim. Place the formed crust into the freezer for 20 minutes while the oven preheats to 375°F (191°C).

When the oven is hot, cook the crust for 10 to 12 minutes, or until lightly golden. Allow it to cool while you prepare the filling.

In a medium saucepan, combine the lemon juice and zest, honey, grass-fed butter and coconut oil to form the filling and cook the mixture over medium low heat until the honey and butter have melted and the filling has slightly thickened, approximately 10 to 12 minutes. Lower the oven temperature to 325°F (163°C) and then pour the filling into the crust. Bake for 25 to 30 minutes or until the filling has set and is no longer jiggly. Allow it to cool for at least 2 hours and serve with fresh fruit.

POACHED PEARS WITH COCONUT CREAM

Yield: 2 pears

While pears may appear fairly unassuming, don't let a plain exterior fool you into believing they're bland or uninteresting. In addition to their fiber-rich profile and subtle sweetness, as well as their contribution to your body's vitamin and mineral levels, there's a secret benefit to pears that might surprise you: They may help you balance your estrogen levels. It's this feature that makes pears a must-have fruit in your hormone-balancing diet. Combine them into a tasty treat by adding a source of healthy fats from coconut cream, and it becomes a poached pear and coconut cream dream!

2 pears

3–4 cups (720–960 ml) water

1 whole star anise

1 cinnamon stick

1 (1-inch [2.5-cm]) piece of ginger, sliced

¼ tsp peppercorns

¼ cup (48 g) + 2 tbsp (24 g) coconut sugar, divided

1 lemon, peel and juice

1 (5.4-oz [160-ml]) can coconut cream (not coconut milk)

1 tbsp (15 ml) agave or honey

Pinch of salt

Peel the pears and slice them in half, and then remove the cores with a melon baller or spoon. Gently place them into a medium-sized, deep saucepan and cover with water—3 to 4 cups (720 to 960 ml) should suffice. Add the star anise, cinnamon stick, ginger, peppercorns, ¼ cup (48 g) of coconut sugar, 2 to 3 long pieces of lemon peel and the juice of the lemon. Bring everything to a very gentle simmer and cook for 10 minutes. If the pears are easily pierced with a fork or knife, they are ready to be removed from the pot with a slotted spoon. Otherwise, continue to cook them for another couple of minutes until they are tender.

Meanwhile, open the can of coconut cream and transfer the cream from the top of the can into a bowl, leaving the liquid behind. Whisk the agave or honey and a small pinch of salt into the coconut cream. Set this aside.

Once the pears have been removed from the poaching liquid, reserve 1 cup (240 ml) of liquid and discard the rest, including the spices. Add 2 tablespoons (24 g) of coconut sugar to the reserved liquid and boil over high heat until reduced to a thick dark syrup. This should take approximately 12 to 15 minutes. Drizzle the pears with the syrup and serve with the coconut cream.

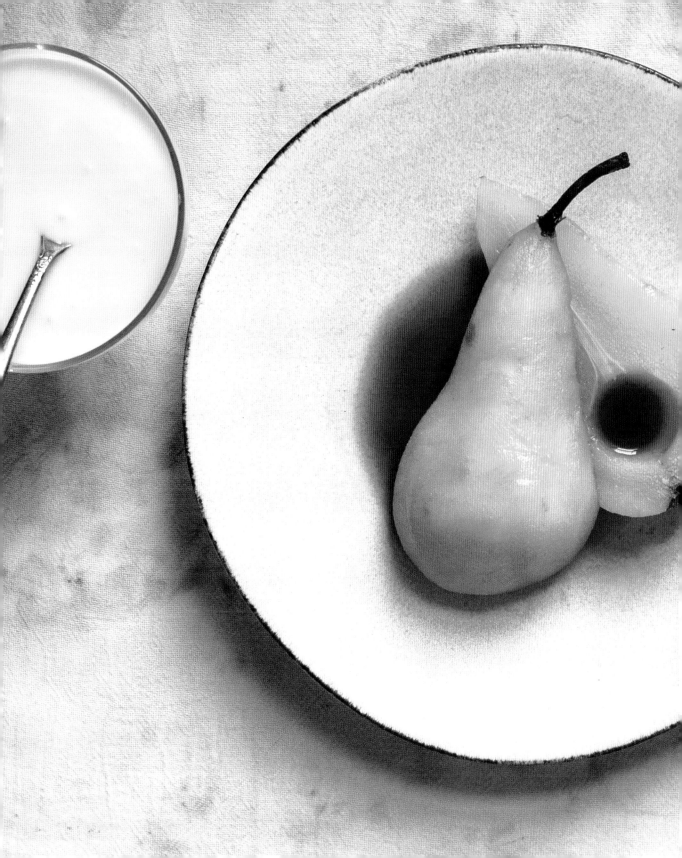

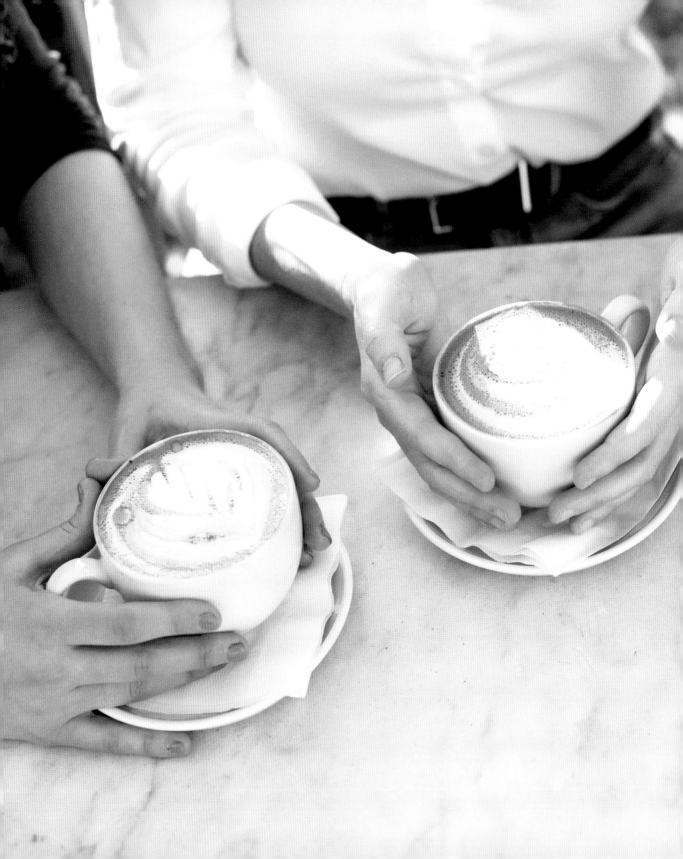

REFERENCES

1. Fuentes, N., & Silveyra, P. (2019). Estrogen receptor signaling mechanisms. Advances in Protein Chemistry and Structural Biology.

2. Large MJ, DeMayo FJ. The regulation of embryo implantation and endometrial decidualization by progesterone receptor signaling. Mol Cell Endocrinol. 2012 Jul 25;358(2):155-65.

3. Snyder, P., et al. Lessons From the Testosterone Trials, Endocrine Reviews, Volume 39, Issue 3, June 2018, 369–386.

4. Klinge, C. M., Clark, B. J., & Prough, R. A. (2018). Dehydroepiandrosterone Research: Past, Current, and Future. Vitamins and Hormones, 1–28.

5. Van der Spek, A. H., Fliers, E., & Boelen, A. (2017). The classic pathways of thyroid hormone metabolism. Molecular and Cellular Endocrinology, 458, 29–38.

6. Tokarz, V. L., MacDonald, P. E., & Klip, A. (2018). The cell biology of systemic insulin function. The Journal of Cell Biology, 217(7), 2273–2289.

7. Ranabir S, Reetu K. Stress and hormones. Indian J Endocrinol Metab. 2011;15(1):18-22.

8. Bull, J.R., Rowland, S.P., Scherwitzl, E.B. et al. Real-world menstrual cycle characteristics of more than 600,000 menstrual cycles. npj Digit. Med. 2, 83 (2019).

9. Reed BG, Carr BR. The Normal Menstrual Cycle and the Control of Ovulation. [Updated 2018 Aug 5]. In: Feingold KR, Anawalt B, Boyce A, et al., editors. Endotext [Internet]. South Dartmouth (MA): MDText.com, Inc.; 2000.

10. McNamara, M., Batur, P., & DeSapri, K. Perimenopause. Annals of Internal Medicine. 2015:162(3):ITC1-ITC16.

11. Jukic AM, Weinberg CR, Baird DD, Wilcox AJ. Lifestyle and reproductive factors associated with follicular phase length. J Womens Health (Larchmt). 2007 Nov;16(9):1340-7.

12. Simitsidellis, I., Saunders, P. T. K., & Gibson, D. A. (2018). Androgens and endometrium: New insights and new targets. Molecular and Cellular Endocrinology, 465, 48–60.

13. Mesen TB, Young SL. Progesterone and the luteal phase: a requisite to reproduction. Obstet Gynecol Clin North Am. 2015;42(1):135-151.

14. Prior JC. Perimenopause: The complex endocrinology of the menopausal transition. Endocr Rev 1998;19:397-428.

15. Santoro N, Brown JR, Adel T et al: Characterization of reproductive hormonal dynamics in the perimenopause. J Clin Endocrinol Metab 81: 1495, 1996.

16. Santoro N: Hormonal changes in the perimenopause. Clinical Consultations in Obstetrics and Gynecology 8: 2, 1996.

17. Kirschbaum C, Schommer N, FederenkoI, et al. Short-term estradiol treatment enhances pituitary-adrenal axis and sympathetic responses to psychosocial stress in healthy young men. J ClinEndocrinol Metab 1996;81:3639-3643.

18. Prior, J. Clearing confusion about perimenopause. BC Medical Journal Vol. 47 No. 10, December 2005.

19. Gottschalk, M., et al. Temporal trends in age at menarche and age at menopause: a population study of 312656 women in Norway, Human Reproduction, 2020. 35(2):464–471.

20. Tanbo, T., & Fedorcsak, P. Can time to menopause be predicted? Acta Obstetricia et Gynecologica Scandinavica. 2021. 100(11):1961-1968.

21. Burger HG, Dudley EC, Robertson DM, Dennerstein L. Hormonal changes in the menopause transition. Recent Prog Horm Res. 2002;57:257-75.

22. G.E. Gillies, S. McArthur, Estrogen actions in the brain and the basis for differential action in men and women: a case for sex-specific medicines, Pharmacol.Rev. 62 (2010) 155–198.

23. Farrell, E. Genitourinary syndrome of menopause. Australian Family Physician, 2017. 46(7):481-484.

24. Shifren, J. Genitourinary Syndrome of Menopause. Clinical Obstetrics and Gynecology, 2018. 61(3):508-516(9).

25. Lephart, E.D., Naftolin, F. Menopause and the Skin: Old Favorites and New Innovations in Cosmeceuticals for Estrogen-Deficient Skin. Dermatol Ther (Heidelb) 11, 53–69 (2021).

26. J. C. Prior (2018) Progesterone for treatment of symptomatic menopausal women, Climacteric, 21:4, 358-365.

27. Johansen, N., et al. The role of testosterone in menopausal hormone treatment. What is the evidence? Acta Obstetricia et Gynecologica Scandinavica. 2020. 99(8):966-969.

28. Kilbreath, K., et al. Prevention of osteoporosis as aconsequence of aromatase inhibitor therapy in postmenopausal women with earlybreast cancer: rationale and design of a randomized controlled trial, Contemp.Clin. Trials 32 (2011) 704–709.

29. Patel, S., et al. (2018). Estrogen: The necessary evil for human health, and ways to tame it. Biomedicine & Pharmacotherapy, 102, 403–411.

30. Santin AP, Furlanetto TW. Role of estrogen in thyroid function and growth regulation. J Thyroid Res. 2011;2011:875125.

31. Cojocaru, M., et al. Manifestations of systemic lupus erythematosus, Mædica 6 (2011) 330–336.

32. Huang, J., et al.Myelin regeneration in multiple sclerosis: targeting endogenous stem cells, Neurotherapeutics 8 (2011) 650–658.

33. Kow, L., & Pfaff, D. Can distinctly different rapid estrogen actions share a common mechanistic step? Hormones and Behavior. 2018.104:156-164.

34. Dumesic D., et al. Scientific Statement on the Diagnostic Criteria, Epidemiology, Pathophysiology, and Molecular Genetics of Polycystic Ovary Syndrome. Endocr. Rev. 2015;36:487–525.

35. Livadas S., et al. Prevalence and impact of hyperandrogenemia in 1218 women with polycystic ovary syndrome. Endocrine. 2014;47:631–638.

36. Rodriguez Paris V, Bertoldo MJ. The Mechanism of Androgen Actions in PCOS Etiology. Med Sci (Basel). 2019;7(9):89. Published 2019 Aug 28. doi:10.3390/medsci7090089.

37. Morgan C., et al. Relationships among plasma dehydroepiandrosterone sulfate and cortisol levels, symptoms of dissociation, and objective performance in humans exposed to acute stress. Arch Gen Psychiatry. 2004 Aug;61(8):819-25.

38. Steriti, R. The Ratio of DHEA or DHEA-S to Cortisol. 2010. Tahoma Clinic.

39. Hardy OT, Czech MP, Corvera S. What causes the insulin resistance underlying obesity?. Curr Opin Endocrinol Diabetes Obes. 2012;19(2):81-87. doi:10.1097/MED.0b013e3283514e13.

40. Gruzdeva O, Borodkina D, Uchasova E, Dyleva Y, Barbarash O. Leptin resistance: underlying mechanisms and diagnosis. Diabetes Metab Syndr Obes. 2019;12:191-198.

41. Chiovato, L., Magri, F. & Carlé, A. Hypothyroidism in Context: Where We've Been and Where We're Going. Adv Ther 36, 47–58 (2019).

42. Watson C, Bulayeva N, Wozniak A, Alyea R. Xenoestrogens are potent activators of nongenomic estrogenic responses. Steroids. 2007;72(2):124-134.

43. Gonsioroski A, Mourikes VE, Flaws JA. Endocrine Disruptors in Water and Their Effects on the Reproductive System. Int J Mol Sci. 2020;21(6):1929. Published 2020 Mar 12. doi:10.3390/ijms21061929.

44. Ajayi, A., & Abraham, K. (2018). Understanding the role of estrogen in the development of benign prostatic hyperplasia. African Journal of Urology, 24(2), 93–97.

45. Vermeulen A, Kaufman JM, Goemaere S, van Pottelberg I. Estradiol in elderly men. Aging Male. 2002;5(2):98-102.

46. Schulster M, Bernie AM, Ramasamy R. The role of estradiol in male reproductive function. Asian J Androl. 2016;18(3):435-440. doi:10.4103/1008-682X.173932.

47. Parida, S., & Sharma, D. (2019). The Microbiome–Estrogen Connection and Breast Cancer Risk. Cells, 8(12), 1642.

48. Ervin, S. M., Li, H., Lim, L., Roberts, L. R., Liang, X., Mani, S., & Redinbo, M. R. (2019). Gut microbiome–derived ⊠-glucuronidases are components of the estrobolome that reactivate estrogens. Journal of Biological Chemistry, jbc. RA119.010950.

49. Baker, J., et al. Estrogen–gut microbiome axis: Physiological and clinical implications. Maturitas. 2017. 103:45-53.

50. Jones, L., et al. The ever-changing roles of serotonin. The International Journal of Biochemistry & Cell Biology. 2020. 125:105776.

51. Zhang, J., Zhang, F., Zhao, C. et al. Dysbiosis of the gut microbiome is associated with thyroid cancer and thyroid nodules and correlated with clinical index of thyroid function. Endocrine 64, 564–574 (2019).

52. Lee, C., et al. Gut microbiome and its role in obesity and insulin resistance. Annals of the New York Academy of Sciences. 2019. 1461(1):37-52.

53. Leonardi, M., Hicks, C., El⊠Assaad, F., El⊠Omar, E., & Condous, G. (2019). Endometriosis and the microbiome: a systematic review. BJOG: An International Journal of Obstetrics & Gynaecology.

54. García-León MÁ, Pérez-Mármol JM, Gonzalez-Pérez R, García-Ríos MDC, Peralta-Ramírez MI. Relationship between resilience and stress: Perceived stress, stressful life events, HPA axis response during a stressful task and hair cortisol. Physiol Behav. (2019) 202:87–93.

55. Sheng, J., et al. The Hypothalamic-Pituitary-Adrenal Axis: Development, Programming Actions of Hormones, and Maternal-Fetal Interactions. Front. Behav. Neurosci. 2021.

56. Baffy G. (2020) General Adaptation Syndrome. In: Zeigler-Hill V., Shackelford T.K. (eds) Encyclopedia of Personality and Individual Differences. Springer, Cham.

57. Nguyen AD, Conley AJ. Adrenal androgens in humans and nonhuman primates: production, zonation and regulation. Endocr Dev. (2008) 13:33–54.

58. Lennartsson AK, Theorell T, Rockwood AL, Kushnir MM, Jonsdottir IH. Perceived stress at work is associated with lower levels of DHEA-S. PLoS One. 2013;8(8):e72460.

59. Różycka, A., Słopień, R., Słopień, A., Dorszewska, J., Seremak-Mrozikiewicz, A., Lianeri, M., … Jagodziński, P. P. (2016). The MAOA, COMT, MTHFR and ESR1 gene polymorphisms are associated with the risk of depression in menopausal women. Maturitas, 84, 42–54.

60. Yin, L., et al. Significant association between methylenetetrahydrofolate reductase gene C677T polymorphism with polycystic ovary syndrome risk. Medicine: January 2020 - Volume 99 - Issue 4 - p e18720

61. Koukoura, O., et al. DNA methylation in endometriosis (Review). Molecular Medicine Reports. 2016. 13(4):2939-2948.

62. Aalaa M, Najmi Varzaneh F, Maghbooli Z, et al. Influence of MTHFR gene variations on perceived stress modification: Preliminary results of NURSE study. Med J Islam Repub Iran. 2017;31:128.

63. Cybulska, A., et al. Depressive Symptoms among Middle-AgedWomen—Understanding the Cause. Brain Sci. 2021, 11, 26.

64. Godar SC, Fite PJ, McFarlin KM, Bortolato M: The role of monoamine oxidase A in aggression: Current translational developments and future challenges. Prog Neuropsychopharmacol Biol Psychiatry 2016;69:90-100.

65. Mikhailova, O., Gulyaeva, L., Prudnikov, A. et al. Estrogen-metabolizing gene polymorphisms in the assessment of female hormone-dependent cancer risk. Pharmacogenomics J 6, 189–193 (2006).

66. Lu, S.-Y., Lin, P., Tsai, W.-R., & Weng, C.-Y. (2019). The Pragmatic Strategy to Detect Endocrine-Disrupting Activity of Xenobiotics in Food. Medicinal Chemistry.

67. Pérez-Miguelsanz J, Vallecillo N, Garrido F, Reytor E, Pérez-Sala D, Pajares MA. Betaine homocysteine S-methyltransferase emerges as a new player of the nuclear methionine cycle. Biochim Biophys Acta Mol Cell Res. 2017 Jul;1864(7):1165-1182.

68. Morio, B., Casas, F., & Pénicaud, L. (2019). Overview of the Cross-Talk Between Hormones and Mitochondria. Mitochondria in Obesity and Type 2 Diabetes, 63–91.

69. Jones, B. G., Sealy, R. E., Penkert, R. R., Surman, S. L., Birshtein, B. K., Xu, B., … Hurwitz, J. L. (2020). From Influenza Virus Infections to Lupus: Synchronous Estrogen Receptor ⍺ and RNA Polymerase II Binding Within the Immunoglobulin Heavy Chain Locus. Viral Immunology.

70. Vom Steeg LG, Vermillion MS, Hall OJ, et al. Age and testosterone mediate influenza pathogenesis in male mice. Am J Physiol Lung Cell Mol Physiol. 2016;311(6):L1234-L1244.

71. Rana SV. Perspectives in endocrine toxicity of heavy metals--a review. Biol Trace Elem Res. 2014 Jul;160(1):1-14.

72. Pollack AZ, Schisterman EF, Goldman LR, et al. Cadmium, lead, and mercury in relation to reproductive hormones and anovulation in premenopausal women. Environ Health Perspect. 2011;119(8):1156-1161.

73. Somppi TL. Non-Thyroidal Illness Syndrome in Patients Exposed to Indoor Air Dampness Microbiota Treated Successfully with Triiodothyronine. Front Immunol. 2017;8:919.

74. Demaegdt H, Daminet B, Evrard A, Scippo ML, Muller M, Pussemier L, Callebaut A, Vandermeiren K. Endocrine activity of mycotoxins and mycotoxin mixtures. Food Chem Toxicol. 2016 Oct;96:107-16.

75. Grassi C, D'Ascenzo M, Torsello A, Martinotti G, Wolf F, Cittadini A, Azzena GB. Effects of 50Hz electromagnetic fields on voltage-gated Ca2+ channels and their role in modulation of neuroendocrine cell proliferation and death. Cell Calcium. 2004;35:307–315.

76. Yaribeygi H, Panahi Y, Sahraei H, Johnston TP, Sahebkar A. The impact of stress on body function: A review. EXCLI J. 2017;16:1057-1072. Published 2017 Jul 21.

77. G.J. Morton, T.H. Meek, M.W. Schwartz.Neurobiology of food intake in health and disease.Nat. Rev. Neurosci., 15 (2014), 367-378.

78. Veronese, N., Reginster, JY. The effects of calorie restriction, intermittent fasting and vegetarian diets on bone health. Aging Clin Exp Res 31, 753–758 (2019).

79. Verkuijl, S.J., Meinds, R.J., Trzpis, M. et al. The influence of demographic characteristics on constipation symptoms: a detailed overview. BMC Gastroenterol 20, 168 (2020).

80. Speranzini LB, Lopasso PP, Laudanna AA. Progesterone, estrogen and pregnancy do not decrease colon myoelectric activity in rats: an in vivo study. Gynecol Obstet Invest. 2008;66:53–58.

81. Baker JM, Al-Nakkash L, Herbst-Kralovetz MM. Estrogen-gut microbiome axis: Physiological and clinical implications. Maturitas. 2017 Sep;103:45-53.

82. Khalif IL, Quigley EM, Konovitch EA, Maximova ID. Alterations in the colonic flora and intestinal permeability and evidence of immune activation in chronic constipation. Dig Liver Dis. 2005;37(11):838–849.

83. Lerner, A., Jeremias, P., & Matthias, T. (2017). Gut-thyroid axis and celiac disease. Endocrine Connections, 6(4), R52–R58. doi:10.1530/ec-17-0021.

84. Liska, D. The Detoxification Enzyme System. Alternative Medicine Review: a Journal of Clinical Therapeutic. 1998. 3(3):187-98.

85. Parcell S. Sulphur in human nutrition and applications in medicine. Altern MedRev. 2002; 7 (1): 22-24.

86. Trickey R (2003). Women's Hormones and the menstrual cycle. Allen & Unwin:Australia.

87. Brody, S. The Relative Health Benefits of Different Sexual Activities. The Journal of Sexual Medicine. 2021. Part 1, 7(4):1336-1361.

88. Heiman JR, Rowland DL, Hatch JP, Gladue BA. Psychophysiological and endocrine responses to sexual arousal in women. Arch Sex Behav. 1991;20:171–86.

89. Gianotten, W., et al. The Health Benefits of Sexual Expression. International Journal of Sexual Health. 2021.

90. Ma, X., et al. The Effect of Diaphragmatic Breathing on Attention, Negative Affect and Stress in Healthy Adults. Front. Psychol. 2017.

91. Lehrer, P., & Woolfolk, R. Principles and Practice of Stress Management, Fourth Edition. The Guilford Press. 2021.

92. Leproult R, Van Cauter E. Role of sleep and sleep loss in hormonal release and metabolism. Endocr Dev. 2010;17:11-21.

93. Klement, R.J., Koebrunner, P.S., Krage, K. et al. Short-term effects of a Paleolithic lifestyle intervention in breast cancer patients undergoing radiotherapy: a pilot and feasibility study. Med Oncol 38, 1 (2021).

94. Patel, S., & Suleria, H. Ethnic and paleolithic diet: Where do they stand in inflammation alleviation? A discussion. Journal of Ethnic Foods. 2017. 4(4):236-241.

95. Bhathena SJ. Relationship between fatty acids and the endocrine system. Biofactors. 2000;13(1-4):35-9.

96. Olivieri, C. Combating insulin resistance with the Paleo diet. The Nurse Practitioner. 2019. 44(2):49-55.

97. Aghasi, M., et al. Dairy intake and acne development: A meta-analysis of observational studies. Clinical Nutrition. 2019. 38(3):1067-1075.

98. Anton, SD, Moehl, K, Donahoo, WT et al. (2018) Flipping the metabolic switch: understanding and applying the health benefits of fasting. Obesity 26, 254–268.

99. Chiofalo B, et al. Fasting as possible complementary approach for polycystic ovary syndrome: Hope or hype? Med Hypotheses. 2017 Aug;105:1-3.

100. Li C, et al. Eight-hour time-restricted feeding improves endocrine and metabolic profiles in women with anovulatory polycystic ovary syndrome. J Transl Med. 2021 Apr 13;19(1):148.

ACKNOWLEDGMENTS

To Our Readers

Thank you for trusting in us to guide you on your health journey. We love to hear your inspiring stories of healing and encourage you to support the ones you love with their health issues as well.

To Our Families

FROM DR. BECKY

Jake, Levi and Liam, you are my world and everything I do is for you. I love you so much. Thank you for being amazing boys and for being my biggest supporters.

Thank you, Mom, for always being by my side and helping me so much with the boys so that I am able to take on as much as I do. You have always been my biggest inspiration to work hard. You are the best role model I could have ever asked for. I love you.

To my sister, Naomi, and my dad, Steve, thank you for continuing to show me the importance of laughter in life. I love you both.

To my best friends Lynn Whitefall, Heidi Larson and Nadine Gallina, no one knows me the way you do or accepts me without any judgement. I love you all so much.

And last but not least, to my favorite partner in crime, Krystal Hohn. Besides being an amazing friend, you are the best partner, in our Health Babes brand and our practice, that anyone could ever ask for. I can't wait to continue creating amazing things together!

FROM DR. KRYSTAL

MY FAMILY

To Chris, my sweet husband, thank you so much for supporting and loving me through all my endeavors. I am so blessed to walk this life with you. Savannah and Declan, everything I do is for you. Thank you for being the best kids a mom could ask for! You are my heart.

Mom, Kyrstin, Sarah and Gary, thank you for being the best family and encouraging me to go after my dreams. Arn and Kathy, thank you for being a core form of support and loving me like your own.

MY FRIENDS

Nicole Brown, you are my person, my rock. Thank you for being my best friend and soul sister. To my New Boston Crew, I love you all with my whole heart and appreciate the life long bond we will always share.

And last but not least, to Becky Campbell, thank you for locking arms with me and building this Health Babes business together. You saw things in me before I could see them in myself, and I love you with my whole heart. Cheers to our amazing future together.

(continued)

ACKNOWLEDGMENTS (CONTINUED)

To Our Publishing Team

Thank you so much Marissa and Will for continuing to let us create content for our readers. You always gave us so much freedom with our vision, and that means the world to us. The entire team at Page Street is so amazing, and we are so grateful to work with you all.

Photography

Thank you, Lindsey Potter, for always capturing such beautiful book covers, lifestyle shots and getting our good sides!

Dani McReynolds, thank you for helping with the beautiful recipe photos. You are truly talented and appreciated.

A Final Note From Us

Working to figure out the best way to support your hormones can be tricky. We know this from working with thousands of women and men in our virtual practice. It is our mission to help as many people as possible get well and live their best lives. We hope that there is enough information in this book to truly help you find what your body needs to thrive. For some, this may be the exact information you have been looking for, and you will do really well just implementing the plan we have laid out in this book. Some may need to work with us or another functional medicine practitioner for some thorough testing to get to the root of the issue. Either way, we are here for you and are so excited to be on this health journey together.

ABOUT THE AUTHORS

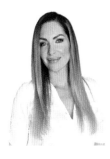

Dr. Becky Campbell

Dr. Becky Campbell is a board-certified doctor of natural medicine who was initially introduced to functional medicine as a patient. She also holds the designation of ADAPT Trained Health Practitioner from the Kresser Institute, the only functional medicine and evolutionary health training company. Dr. Campbell is also a certified Wahls Protocol Health Practitioner. She struggled with many of the same issues her patients struggle with today, and she has made it her mission to help patients all around the world with her virtual practice. Dr. Becky Campbell is the founder of Dr.BeckyCampbell.com, the host of The Health Babes Podcast and author of *The 30-Day Thyroid Reset Plan, The 4-Phase Histamine Reset Plan, Long Hauler Road Map: A Guide to Recovery from Histamine Intolerance, MCAS and Long Hauler Syndrome* and *Fifty-One Low Histamine Air Fryer Recipes*. She has been featured on multiple online publications like Mindbodygreen, Bustle, PopSugar, *People* magazine, *Men's Health, InStyle* magazine and more. She has been a guest on the Mind Pump Podcast, Bulletproof Radio, The Genius Life Podcast and many others as a thyroid/hormone health & Histamine Intolerance expert. Dr. Campbell specializes in Histamine Intolerance, Thyroid disease, hormone health and autoimmune disease and hopes to help others regain their lives as functional medicine helped her regain hers.

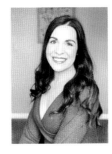

Dr. Krystal Hohn

Dr. Krystal Hohn is passionate about helping people experience optimal health through functional medicine. She works with people of all ages focusing on identifying and addressing the underlying causes of a health setback or disease, rather than just suppressing symptoms. She is a board-certified doctor of natural medicine (DNM), and also earned her doctorate in Chiropractic at Life University in Marietta, GA (DC). She also holds the designation of ADAPT Trained Health Practitioner from Kresser Institute, the only functional medicine and evolutionary health training company. Dr. Krystal has also trained extensively under Chris Kresser, M.S., LAc, a globally recognized leader in the fields of ancestral health and integrative medicine.

Dr. Hohn and Dr. Campbell work together virtually with patients from all over the world. They are also the hosts of the popular Health Babes Podcast and Health Babes brand.

Where to Find The Health Babes

For one-on-one consultations and free resources: https://drbeckycampbell.com/

Podcast: The Health Babes Podcast

Instagram: @healthbabespodcast @drbeckycampbell @drkrystalhohn

Online Program Coming Soon!

INDEX

prostate, enlarged, 36
prostate cancer, 30
protein powders, 63
proteins, 56, 63
pudding
    Avocado Chia Pudding, 146
    Baked Pumpkin Pudding, 142
Pumpkin Pudding, Baked, 142
pumpkin seeds: Roasted Salmon
    Salad, 106

Q

quercetin, 129

R

radio waves, 50
radishes: Lamb Tacos with Paleo
    Tzatziki, 117
rapeseed oil, 65
receptors, 15–16
red wine, 65
refined foods, 68
relaxation, 59
restaurant food, 67
restrictive eating, 52–53
reverse T3, 44
romaine lettuce: Chicken Caesar Kale
    Salad, 102

S

safflower oil, 65, 68
salad dressings. See dressings
salads, 71
    Avocado & Citrus Salad, 134
    Beet & Orange Salad, 133
    Chicken Caesar Kale Salad, 102
    Herby Tomato & Cucumber
        Salad, 137
    Italian Seared Beef Salad, 113
    Roasted Salmon Salad, 106
    Savory Steak Salad, 97
Salmon Salad, Roasted, 106
sauces, processed, 68
sausage
    Huevos Rancheros, 86
    Sausage, Apple and Kale-Stuffed
        Butternut Squash, 126
    Swiss Chard Crepes, 77

seafood
    Roasted Salmon Salad, 106
    Shrimp Fajitas, 125
seasonings, 68
seed oils, 65, 67, 68
seeds, 67
    Avocado & Citrus Salad, 134
    Roasted Salmon Salad, 106
    Savory Seed Porridge, 81
selenium, 40
serotonin, 40, 47, 55
sex
    benefits of, 57
    pain during, 28
sex drive
    low, 21, 22, 28, 30, 35, 54
    perimenopause and, 21
    testosterone and, 21, 28
sex hormones, 18, 44, 48, 49
    See also estrogen; progesterone;
        testosterone
Shallot Vinaigrette, 106
SHBG, 31, 64
Shrimp Fajitas, 125
side dishes
    Avocado & Citrus Salad, 134
    Beet & Orange Salad, 133
    Herby Tomato & Cucumber
        Salad, 137
    Roasted Asparagus with Cashew
        Sauce, 138
    Roasted Carrots with Creamy
        Herb Dressing, 141
singing, 59
skin, 28, 32, 64
sleep, 60
sleep disturbances, 23, 24, 27, 28, 34,
    55
snap peas, 67
sodas, 68
soups, 71
    Chicken Tortilla Soup, 114
    Creamy Broccoli Soup, 94
    Roasted Carrot & Fennel Soup
        with Chicken, 110
    Turkey Meatball Soup, 130
soybean oil, 65, 68
soy sauce, 68
Spaghetti Squash & Meatballs, 122
sperm, 21
spices, 63

spinach
    Savory Seed Porridge, 81
    Spaghetti Squash & Meatballs,
        122
    Spinach & Shallot Omelet, 73
    Turkey Meatball Soup, 130
sprouts: Avocado & Citrus Salad, 134
squash
    Sausage, Apple and Kale-Stuffed
        Butternut Squash, 126
    Spaghetti Squash & Meatballs,
        122
Steak Salad, Savory, 97
stress
    chronic, 32–33, 43–44
    cortisol and, 19, 32–33, 43, 44,
        46, 48
    DHEA and, 18, 32–33, 43, 44
    impacts of, 43–44
    management, 59–60
    men and, 36
    MTHFR gene and, 46
sugar, 64, 65, 68
sugar peas, 67
sulfur, 56, 89
sunflower seed oil, 65, 68
sweeteners, 68
sweet potatoes
    Paleo Chili, 121
    Sweet Potato Hashbrown Cups,
        85
Swiss Chard Crepes, 77

T

T3 hormone, 18, 29, 40, 43, 44, 54
T4 hormone, 18, 29, 40, 43, 44, 54
Tabbouleh with Chicken Breast, 101
tacos
    Breakfast Tacos, 74
    Cauliflower Rice Taco Bowl, 98
    Lamb Tacos with Paleo Tzatziki,
        117
tamari, 68
Tart, Lemon, 149
taurine, 56
tea, 67
tequila, 65
testes, 16

testosterone, 18, 48
    decline in, 28, 44
    elevated, 31–32
    functions of, 28
    imbalances, 36
    inflammation and, 49
    menopause and, 28
    menstrual cycle and, 20, 21
thymus, 16
thyroid, 16, 30, 40, 43, 49, 50, 60
thyroid-binding globulin (TBG), 29
thyroid hormones, 18, 29, 40, 43, 44, 48, 54, 69
thyroid imbalances, 34
TNF gene, 45
tomatoes
    Breakfast Tacos, 74
    Chicken Caesar Kale Salad, 102
    Chicken Tortilla Soup, 114
    Egg Bites, 82
    Herby Tomato & Cucumber Salad, 137
    Mediterranean Skillet Chicken, 129
    Paleo Chili, 121
    Savory Steak Salad, 97
    Spaghetti Squash & Meatballs, 122
    Swiss Chard Crepes, 77
    Tabbouleh with Chicken Breast, 101
tortillas
    Breakfast Tacos, 74
    Chicken Tortilla Soup, 114
    Huevos Rancheros, 86
    Lamb Tacos with Paleo Tzatziki, 117
toxins, 49–50, 56, 57, 60
TRH, 43
triglycerides, 33
TSH, 43, 44
Turkey Meatball Soup, 130
Tzatziki, 117

U
urinary tract, 28
urinary tract infections (UTIs), 28
uterine cancer, 30
uterine fibroids, 30, 40

V
vagina, menopause and, 26, 28
vagus nerve, 59
vanilla extract, 64
vegetables, 61
    See also specific vegetables
    brassica, 89
    cruciferous, 61
    pickled, 105
vinegar, 67
viral infections, 49
vitamin B12, 113
vitamin C, 133, 134, 149
vodka, 65

W
walnuts: Beet & Orange Salad, 133
water, 55, 57
weight gain, 40, 52, 54
    cortisol and, 19
    during perimenopause, 23, 24
weight loss, 52, 69
weight management, 60, 69
whole foods, 61
wine, 65
women
    fasting and, 71
    hormone fluctuations and, 34–35
    immune system and, 49
wrinkles, 28

X
X chromosome, 47
xenobiotics, 47
xenoestrogens, 36, 45

Z
zinc, 40, 65